Overcoming Anxiety

DAVID HAZARD

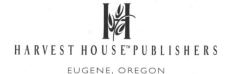

HARVEST HOUSE™PUBLISHERS

EUGENE, OREGON

Cover by Left Coast Design, Portland, Oregon

Advisory

Readers are advised to consult with their physician or other medical practitioner before implementing the suggestions that follow.

This book is not intended to take the place of sound medical advice or to treat specific maladies. Neither the author nor the publisher assumes any liability for possible adverse consequences as a result of the information contained herein.

OVERCOMING ANXIETY
Copyright © 2003 by David Hazard
Published by Harvest House Publishers
Eugene, Oregon 97402

Library of Congress Cataloging-in-Publication Data

Hazard, David.
      Overcoming anxiety / David Hazard.
          p. cm. — (Healthy body, healthy soul series)
      ISBN 0-7369-1194-4 (pbk.)
      1. Anxiety—Religious aspects—Christianity. I. Title. II. Series.
      BT731.5.H39 2003
      616.85'22306—dc21   2003004003

Printed in the United States of America.

    03   04   05   06   07   08   09   10   11   / BP-CF /   10   9   8   7   6   5   4   3   2   1

Contents

Healthy Body, Healthy Soul

The *Healthy Body, Healthy Soul* series is being developed to meet the needs of everyday men, women, and children, as reflected in three important trends in healthcare.

The first is a return to a *whole-person approach to health.*

Scientists are rediscovering what ancient physicians knew. The body, mind, and spirit are amazingly interconnected, and they work together—*in sympathy*—with each other. This ancient understanding—that we are integrated beings, not separate in our parts—is even reflected in the words of the psalmist, who observed that his physical being and his inner being (the Hebrew word encompasses *mind, emotions,* and *spirit*) were carefully *"knit together in my mother's womb...fearfully and wonderfully made...woven together"* (Psalm 139:13-15).

The interconnectedness of our whole being can present us with a serious problem. When one aspect of our being is damaged—say our mind or emotions—it can have negative repercussions throughout our whole being. We experience what is called a *psychosomatically based* illness. Many studies in the scientific community, in the fields of psychology and medicine, have proven this to be true. But that's the unhappy news.

The good news? Because we are interconnected—body, mind, and spirit—when we create health in one aspect of our being it can have amazing benefits for the whole person. For example, the healthcare community has recently rediscovered the overall benefits of simple, regular physical activity, whether from an exercise program or good old sweat-raising hard work. It's a proven fact that people who increase their physical activity regularly not only experience lowered cholesterol and a greatly reduced risk of heart disease...they also think sharper, experience less depression (or overcome it if they've had it) and more of the brighter moods, *and* have a more buoyant outlook on life. In short, they become healthier in body, mind, and soul.

The second important trend is the movement toward *self care.* Today's healthcare consumers are the most educated in history. They're also more willing to assume responsibility for their health than their ancestors, who were generally more passive in relegating the care of their body, soul, and spirit to "experts." We know that most of these experts focused on their own areas of knowledge. What they *don't* know can hurt us. It's the extremely rare expert who is aware of all our options. And knowing all our options can be critical when it comes to treating health conditions.

For this reason, I believe it's crucial that each one of us become the "captain" of our own healthcare team. At the same time, I believe it's important that we have healthcare professionals—be they doctors, psychologists, chiropractors, nutritionists, or others—as our trusted advisers. But in the end, *you and I* are the best advocates for our own needs. When it comes down to it, our needs, experiences, observations, and desires count the most. And as the great Rabbi Simon Maimonides put it, "If I am not for me, then who is for me?"

Finally, we as a culture are rapidly trending toward the use of natural remedies and complementary therapies. We are using these means of treating sickness, or staying well, in two ways: *along with* traditional western medical protocols, or *in place of* them.

Our discoveries about, for instance, the pharmaceuticals we're using is just one reason for this cultural swing. Many of us have learned that, though our drugs can combat illnesses effectively, they can also have serious side effects. They can also encourage a psychological dependence—a *"just give me a pill for it"* mentality—when taking a medication will only treat symptoms, but not resolve the real root of the health problem.

Fortunately, as we've become more educated and self-motivated, we've been rediscovering natural remedies and therapies used by our ancestors, sometimes for millenia.

All told, we as a culture are waking up to an important truth: Taking the responsibility of our own healthcare, and finding out what therapies work best *for us*—including natural remedies and therapies—gives us the best chance of recovery from any health condition we suffer. Today, countless testimonials are proving this to be true. This is an important awakening.

And this is where *Healthy Body, Healthy Soul* books come in. Each one offers practical strategies for the care of body, mind, and soul that are proven to work. The strategies found in this book can help if you are suffering from generalized anxiety or anxiety disorders by helping you—

> • *learn mental stress relief techniques to release anxious thoughts*
>
> • *discover spiritual practices that restore deep-soul peace*
>
> • *correct your diet, if certain foods, food additives, and even eating habits are contributing to your anxiety*
>
> • *ease into a plan for physical activities that are unbeatable "mood-lifters"*
>
> • *learn about natural supplements, and how to use them effectively*

As you create the anxiety-relief strategy that works for you, my wish is that you will experience good health…in body and soul.

David Hazard
Founder of The New Nature Institute

1

Freedom Is Possible

Both generalized anxiety and anxiety disorders have plagued my family for several generations. For that reason, of all the books in the *Healthy Body, Healthy Soul* series, this one comes from a place closest to where I live every day.

Looking back to my grandparents' generation, it's now apparent that at least one of them suffered such acute anxiety it's likely his alcoholism was the result of an attempt to self-medicate the awful feelings that, otherwise, consumed his waking hours. Listening to family members reminisce, the signs of anxiety disorder were there—but in those days nobody knew what an anxiety disorder was.

In the generation that followed—that of my parents—the medical community was still behind the curve on such things and uncontrollable anxiety forced one relative to drop out of high school.

In my generation, anxiety affected me as a teenager when I suffered from a disorder that caused severe depression and affected my ability to eat. As you may imagine, this had drastic health consequences.

At present, two of my three children suffer with Obsessive-Compulsive Disorder (one of the major forms of anxiety disorder). Two relatives on my wife's side of the family also suffer from anxiety disorders. Again, as little as 20 years ago, the drastic effects of anxiety were just becoming known, and "anxiety disorder" was just becoming an official diagnosis.

What's sobering is that we are not *that* unusual. According to the Anxiety Disorder Association of America, more than 13 percent of adults—about 19 million people—suffer from some form of anxiety disorder that is interrupting their lives. Even allowing for the under-reporting of such things as anxiety disorders in the past (when "generalized anxiety" and "anxiety disorder" were not official diagnoses), experts believe we are experiencing a rapid rise in cases of generalized anxiety and anxiety disorders in our culture.

Why this is so—whether the problem lies with our intense pace of life, our diet, food additives, changes in the environment, or other factors—is still open to investigation. We just don't know.

The Torment of Anxiety

What we can say for sure is that anxiety and anxiety disorders make life *miserable*, a true torment.

To begin with, there is the psychological stress of the anxiety itself—that uncomfortable, terrible sense we carry that *something bad is about to happen.* And though we're not sure *what*, we sense that we're powerless to stop it.

Physically we're in "fight or flight" mode, ready for the assault we believe to be on its way. Two "orders" are sent throughout our body. The first order commands one set of glands to produce an abundance of the "stress" hormones. Our body tenses as these hormones pump into our muscles. Blood pressure elevates. Breathing gets shallow, reducing our oxygen supply.

The second "order" goes out to a set of glands that produces what we might think of as "peace-time" hormones—those needed for routine bodily functions, for immunity and the repair of cells and tissues damaged in the normal course of living. The order says, "Slow or stop production until the assault is over." Our body is in a state of "high alert." We feel edgy. Sleeping is difficult. We may be headachy. If you're a woman, your normal monthly cycle may become irregular or even cease.

But that's not all.

Emotionally, we're edgy, easily irritated, not happy. Our ability to relate to other people suffers. *Mentally,* we're preoccupied, leaving little energy for focusing on other people…let alone focusing on free, creative thinking. When we're under assault, we can't focus on bettering our own lives and careers. *Spiritually,* we feel alone, cut-off from the nurture, support, or wisdom available from other people…or even from God. Relationships suffer, as the people in our lives get weary of the tension and limitations our anxieties force upon them.

As if that's not bad enough, a *second level of anxiety* can kick in.

Even on good days we can limit ourselves because we're afraid a bout with anxiety *might* occur. As one businessman put it, "I experienced panic attacks two different times while I was traveling on business. Suddenly I was gripped with terror. My heart was racing. I was sweating bullets. And I thought I was going to die. Being alone, thousands of miles from home and feeling so overwhelmed by anxiety was horrible. After that, every time another business trip came up just the *thought* of it made me anxious. So I started resisting business travel. Because of that, my work and my career suffered."

Without intervention, anxiety spreads from one facet of life to another. The trap becomes tighter. Life closes in. We're unable to live free…to enjoy the life of simple peace and happiness we long for.

What Type of Anxiety Do You Experience?

Yes, there is something of an epidemic of anxiety and anxiety disorders in our culture. In one way it helps to know we're not alone. But for those of us who suffer with these life-limiting conditions the important issue is, *What can I do about it? How can I find relief?*

Overcoming Anxiety offers a whole-person approach, using natural remedies and alternative therapies to help you escape from the awful symptoms of generalized anxiety and to manage panic attacks and the symptoms of anxiety disorders. The strategies offered here really work. Before we go further, though, we need to make some crucial distinctions. It's important to understand that there are differences between *generalized anxiety, panic attacks,* and *anxiety disorders*—and in the ways they're treated.

Compare these true-life cases.

Beth

Her best friends jokingly teased her about being "the nervous type." Her husband sometimes got annoyed, but usually tried to encourage her through the rougher days. "You worry about *everything*. You make a hobby out of it," he joked. But the anxiety Beth felt much of the time was no laughing matter.

Most days started out okay. But, by mid-morning the symptoms kicked in just after she began her workday, which included managing her home-based business, keeping up with the kids' schedules, and taking care of the house. Once she'd been good at this, but now, suddenly, she'd experience a sense of being overwhelmed.

From there it was all downhill. Emotionally, it was as if the chaos she felt inside spread out to take in the whole world. Everything asked of her felt like too much. Some days, mentally, it seemed like her circuits were jamming. She felt confused, unable to do anything other than the simplest tasks. Sometimes she'd even find herself moving in slow motion, as if just thinking about walking from one room to the other was labor. Physically, her stomach would tense, her breathing would go shallow, and she'd feel shaky.

On the worst days, she could rock between moments where she experienced a deep sense of well-being…and then suddenly find herself on the edge of a precipice, feeling that if she let go she would start crying or screaming. Visits with several healthcare professionals failed to reveal a cause.

Beth's problem didn't seem to be related to her monthly cycle. Psychologically, she had no "deep wounds" left over from some traumatic past event. But now her self-esteem was suffering blow after blow. Every time she experienced an episode, she'd privately bash herself, saying, "What is *wrong* with you? Stop acting like such a weak little *basket case*." Her self-confidence was all but gone.

Beth was experiencing some of the classic symptoms of *generalized anxiety*. As counseling eventually revealed, her anxiety had an *external trigger.* In her case, Beth was overwhelmed with too much responsibility and too many "To Do" lists. Before she knew what was happening, her sense of being mentally overwhelmed caused her to physically tense up. This, in turn, sent out the signals to her hormonal system. In time she developed a sort of hair trigger. Her anxiety became "generalized" in that anything, everything, or sometimes nothing at all, could trigger the release of stress hormones. Then even plain old living seemed like too much. The smallest task was too big.

"It felt like I was fighting a war on a dozen battlefronts all at once," Beth says. "I got help from a counselor at first. It helped to talk to someone. But in fact I had to learn how to manage my life all over again. I got a lot of help by learning some simple mental and spiritual stress relief strategies. I also had to make some adjustments in my personal relationships. These strategies changed my life."

Compare Beth's condition with that of Matt, Carman, Alan, or Jayne, who suffer from *anxiety disorders.*

Matt

There were certain words Matt could not hear spoken. If he did, he'd have to tap his fingers together 300 times—discreetly, of course, so no one would see and ask what he was doing. Secretly, he was having to "undo" what the forbidden words had done.

There were things Matt could not touch or be touched by. Pens or pencils, for instance. At the end of a school day, after *having* to touch writing utensils all day, he'd come home and go through rituals to "undo" what touching a pen or pencil had done.

There were doorways Matt could not go through. This included the main doorway into his family's apartment. Many days, before or after going through the doorway he'd have to stop and make a circle on the floor with his toe…or turn his head to one side and count to 100…or he'd have to do some other ritual. Whatever his mind demanded of him to "undo" the effects of the forbidden thing he'd just done was always changing. He only knew he *had* to do it or something terrible would happen.

Matt's self-esteem was taking a terrible beating. He knew what he was doing made no sense, but he couldn't stop himself. "I'm an idiot," he'd tell himself, mercilessly. "A psycho. A total basket case." And his social relationships suffered immensely from his compulsions. "If anyone sees me doing these stupid things they'll think I'm a freak." So he began avoiding his friends and tucking his secret deeper inside. At home, he'd become upset if someone said one of the "forbidden words" or interrupted him in the middle of one of his rituals, which, of course, happened all the time. Family life became hellish.

Matt was experiencing symptoms of one of the major anxiety disorders—in this case, Obsessive-Compulsive Disorder (OCD). OCD, like other anxiety disorders, has an *internal trigger*. OCD is thought to result from a physiological condition in which the neurotransmitter chemicals in the brain are not functioning properly. The healthcare establishment's current treatment for most anxiety disorders involves the use of certain prescription drugs and behavior modification therapy.

Carman

Carman *needed* to blink his eyes. Sometimes he *needed* to clear his throat. Sometimes he *needed* to tighten his facial muscles into a grimace. It was a compulsion that felt as strong and automatic as a hiccup.

Carman was experiencing a version of anxiety disorder which was, in the past, referred to as a "nervous tic." In fact, it is a condition associated with Tourette's Syndrome, which has become known popularly for one of its more flamboyant, possible symptoms, which is a sudden outburst of angry, insulting, or profane words.

At present, the healthcare community treats this particular disorder primarily with pharmaceuticals and some behavior therapy.

Alan

In college, Alan was one of the most outgoing guys you'd ever meet. He played sports and belonged to a service fraternity. And on his first job after graduation he became the shining star of client relations, hopping on planes to fly all over the country and solve customer crises.

One evening, at an outdoor concert, Alan began to feel shaky. Not long after, at his son's soccer game, he had a terrible feeling something bad was going to happen. Two months later, Alan had trouble leaving the house even for necessary reasons, like driving to work.

Alan was suffering from a form of anxiety that presents itself in the form of a *phobia*. For Alan, it was *agoraphobia*, a fear of being out in open places. In his case, there was no traumatic emotional event at its root.

One characteristic of phobias is that they can change over time, or they can multiply. One kind of fear may disappear, only to be replaced by another. Or the original fear will be joined by others until, over time, the sufferer is plagued by a host of phobias.

In Alan's case, as in most others, *exposure therapy* was necessary. Under the care of a professional, Alan was taught to expose himself to places and experiences that caused him anxiety, as he learned how to confront the uncomfortable feelings they caused or to distract himself by turning to pastimes he found positive and pleasant.

Jayne

Jayne had always been thin. As a little girl, she'd been a great eater. Not picky.

Sometime in the middle of her sophomore year in high school, friends noticed that Jayne barely ate any lunch. Through her clothing, you could see her shoulder joints protruding, and her cheeks were sunken.

A therapist was able to peg the onset of Jayne's problem—an anxiety disorder, in her case, *anorexia*—to the traumatic event of her parents' divorce. The anxiety Jayne felt in the pit of her stomach when her family split apart was beyond her control. The physical sensation she got when she ate was not. If she could just keep *any*

℞

IF YOU ARE SUFFERING FROM ACUTE ANXIETY OR AN ANXIETY DISORDER

～

If you're having anxiety problems, it is crucial for you to get help from a physician, psychologist, or psychiatrist to establish an accurate diagnosis.

Certain physical conditions can cause anxiety, such as high blood pressure, thyroid deficiencies, and more serious disorders of the brain chemistry, to name a few. These require professional assistance. A healthcare professional can help determine whether an illness or disorder is behind the uncomfortable feelings you're suffering.

Second, it's possible that your condition will require you to use a prescription medication. In cases where even generalized anxiety is severe enough, you may sometimes need fast intervention in the form of a prescription drug. And if you're experiencing an anxiety disorder you will most certainly benefit initially from the use of pharmaceuticals. Though their effectiveness and side effects need to be carefully monitored, do not be hesitant to use medications when they can benefit you.

Behavior-modification therapy may also be helpful in treating your anxiety or anxiety disorder. Usually, this involves "exposure therapy," which is learning how to encounter the object, person, or situation that triggers anxiety, and doing so in a controlled (safe) environment. This is helpful in learning how to calm the anxious feelings with rational (nonanxious) thinking.

Bottom Line: Even if your goal is a totally natural treatment program, complementary treatments, including the natural remedies and therapies found in this book, *can* be carefully blended with traditional healthcare practices to create a healing program that works for you.

Let good sense rule.

sensation out of that traumatized center-place of her being, everything would feel okay.

What complicated things for Jayne was that she did get very hungry. And so she ate. But now, eating made her feel not just physically uncomfortable in her stomach…but emotionally uncomfortable, too. At some point, the simple little trick she'd learned to keep from feeling uncomfortable had taken on a life of its own. Her anorexia had become *bulimia,* as well. She couldn't break the cycle of eating in tiny amounts, then forcing herself to purge what she'd eaten. Of course this wreaked havoc with her brain and body chemistry. Her emotions and thinking were in a scramble of anxiety.

At the present time, eating disorders such as Jayne's are treated by the traditional healthcare community with counseling in a caring, supportive environment, and at times with the use of medications.

Whether you are suffering generalized anxiety or an anxiety disorder you can benefit greatly by finding the natural remedies and treatments in this book that work for you. They can be used to complement and boost the effectiveness of the help you get from a healthcare professional. It may even be possible for you to create a whole-person program, personalized to your needs, that will help you take control of the anxiety or anxiety disorder that traps you now and free you to be at peace and experience the amazing joy of living again.

A basic principle of natural healing is that
body and soul were made to work together.
To get well, we need balance.

You Need a Plan That Benefits You—Body and Soul

Overcoming Anxiety, like the other books in the *Healthy Body, Healthy Soul* series, is written with a certain strategy in mind. We'll begin by looking at interior issues that can lie at the root of anxiety. Many times healing comes from dealing with mental, emotional, or spiritual conflicts. These stressors may lie at the root of the anxiety problem, or they may be strong contributing factors. What we need to learn are the mental and spiritual practices that restore health to our inner being.

Then we'll look at natural strategies for dealing with anxiety that comes from physiologically based disorders. We'll discuss foods that can trigger anxiety and create a new and delicious diet from foods that help keep your mood peaceful and even. We'll find the best anxiety-busting physical workout for you, whether you're into "minimal exercise, please" or you're the kind of person who wants to go "all out."

Finally, you'll get the most up-to-date information on potent vitamins, herbs, and other natural supplements that can help release anxiety.

At a more fundamental level, though, finding our path to freedom from the anxiety that plagues us begins with taking the right mindset.

Step 1: Recognize You Are a Whole Person

You are an amazingly interconnected being, with a soul and a body. Either they are working against each other or they're working together.

Anxiety can be a symptom that may be telling you several important aspects of your life—inwardly or outwardly—need attention and care. And the nature of anxiety is that the dis-ease it causes *will* spread from one aspect of your being to another, affecting you physically, mentally, and spiritually.

One of the most basic principles of natural healing is that the body and soul were made to work together. When one aspect of our being is suffering, our whole being will eventually suffer. The good news is that as you remedy each area of life in which you're suffering you begin to create *a climate of wellness* that generates healing throughout your whole being—a healing balance.

Step 2: Become the Captain of Your Own Healthcare Team

No one benefits more than you, when you take charge of your own care. When we take an active role in seeking the help we need we are most likely to get well. Too many of us are passive where our health and well-being are concerned. Experts and professionals are an important part of our healthcare team. But we are the only ones who know how various treatments help us, hurt us, or do nothing at all. We are also the only ones who know the wide-ranging effects of anxiety or an anxiety disorder, therefore we are the only ones who can say, "This treatment helped me get better in one way, but anxiety is still hurting me in this other aspect of my life."

I am speaking from personal experience: If you suffer from anxiety, you need to take the time—and it does take time—to examine *each* aspect of your being carefully. Do the kind of careful inventory that will tell you where you're struggling, impaired, and need real help.

For this reason, it's important that you read *every* chapter of this book and avoid the temptation to flip to the solutions you think you'd like to try first. (You'll find the chapter on natural supplements later in the book because it's important for you to consider strategies that focus on lifestyle change *before* you reach for the vitamin and herb bottles for "quick and easy" solutions.) And if you're thinking of *skipping* certain chapters altogether (for instance, the one on exercise!), read those chapters *twice.* They probably offer the strategies that will benefit you the most.

Begin Today

As you may be gathering, *seeking balanced solutions* and *taking personal responsibility* are fundamental keys in taking the whole-person approach to natural healing. As you find the various natural remedies that work for you, you will begin to restore balance throughout your whole being—body, mind, and spirit. Continue to take charge of your recovery. Make these strategies part of your life. You'll find yourself becoming mentally sharper, spiritually more full of life, physically stronger, and more resilient...*and*, best of all, you'll feel the grip of anxiety letting go.

Today, begin to follow the healing path that will lead you out of the life-limiting trap of anxiety and anxiety disorders. Without a doubt you can find the deep sense of peace, well-being, and confidence your anxiety has taken from you. You can take back the life that's yours...a *whole life.*

2

Getting the "Big Picture"

Virtually everyone experiences anxiety at some time in their life. But we need to make an important distinction. Anxiety is a normal human response when we encounter something that threatens our well-being. Being away from home and suddenly remembering you left the stove on...having your teenage daughter out way past curfew and no phone call...hearing that there will be job cutbacks at work—those experiences trigger anxiety in otherwise emotionally steady people.

But for those who suffer chronic anxiety, fear—even bordering on panic—occurs more and more often, triggered by less and less threatening events. At this point, you cross the line from "normal" anxiety to what healthcare professionals recognize as unhealthy *generalized anxiety*. At this point, treatment becomes necessary.

And then there are those, like Mark, whose anxiety comes without warning, attached to no specific triggering events. For these people, the sudden onset of anxiety—in his case, *panic attacks*—can be as perplexing as it is devastating.

"The first time I experienced a panic attack," says Mark as he shifts uneasily in his chair, "I was on a business trip, thousands of miles from home, in a foreign culture for the first time...and it was the dead of night. I'd been exhausted when I fell asleep and woke suddenly in pitch-dark. I didn't exactly 'wake up.' It was as if a horse had kicked me in the back, jolting me upright from the bed. My heart was racing, pounding in my chest, my neck, my face, my scalp....My chest felt compressed and my windpipe seemed to be blocked, preventing me from sucking air into my lungs.

"The involuntary muscles in my diaphragm kicked in and I started to breathe. But that only made things worse. It was like the time when I was a kid and froze my hands making ice balls to throw at cars. 'Numb' doesn't hurt, but as your skin thaws and the feelings sizzle into your nerve-endings again...*I was shouting, with the intense pain.* Breathing made me feel as if I were drowning.

"The words 'anxiety' or 'panic' don't come close to describing the actual feelings that ripped through me until dawn. That same awful jolt kept hitting me in shock waves. A tornado of mental images flooded my head—awful pictures of my wife and two young sons...dead. Images of myself...dead. And at the same time a black chasm kept opening in the floor of my soul. I imagined myself dropping into a cold, black underground...lost and abandoned."

Maybe you've never experienced a panic attack, as Mark has, but his description of it brings up one universal characteristic of anxiety in all its various forms: Anxiety is an uncomfortable sense that, to a greater or lesser degree, *engulfs* us. Depending on its intensity, it builds and blocks out more and more of our *other* feelings, and clouds our thoughts. It darkens our inner landscape the way thick storm clouds slowly cover the sky and smother the ground in deep shadow. When the tension of anxiety is severe enough—like when we suffer a traumatic shock, or a panic attack, or an anxiety disorder—it billows up and fills our whole "inner horizon." We are swallowed up by the overwhelming feelings of anxiety.

In our desire to overcome anxiety—whether in the form of panic attacks like Mark's or general anxiety like Beth's in Chapter 1—we can be better equipped if we understand the "big picture"—and the "trail" of choices we can make that empowers us to walk free of anxiety and live a healthy, peaceful, balanced life.

First, You Need Perspective

Getting the "big picture" means clearly understanding the steps that will help you turn anxious impulses into calm responses. It means understanding that we have choices to make—to let anxiety engulf us, or to learn how to resist it and use its energy to activate a positive response. It means getting perspective.

Our anxious behavior is not as "automatic" as most of us think. Anxiety *feels* like a force that strikes "instantly" and "forces" us to react the way we do. The truth is, *anxious impulses* may come at us out of nowhere, but our *anxious response* is really a pattern of behavior we've formed to "shake off" the uncomfortable feeling that's juicing through our bodies.

Getting the big picture helps us understand how anxiety becomes that terrible force that overwhelms us and crowds out our ability to function freely and at peace. Unless we take time to understand how anxiety works, we're likely to seek relief in one or two strategies that offer immediate relief only to find that anxiety abates temporarily. When we do that, we doom ourselves to limping through life, merely managing each episode of anxiety but never really escaping it.

Taking time to understand ourselves, on the other hand, can show several important things: *First,* the "path" of our own anxiety—where and how it begins and how its energy grows. *Second,* how important it is to address *every* aspect of our life—body, mind, and spirit. *Third,* how to create the most effective personal strategy to escape anxiety's grip.

Whether you are dealing with chronic generalized anxiety, an anxiety disorder, or panic attacks, getting the big picture can help you begin to build a personal strategy. That's because it will create a foundation of calm objectivity, a "steady base" of consciousness, from which you can learn to turn anxious energy in a healthy direction.

Working through the steps in this chapter will help you begin to use objective thinking and strategizing to take charge of emotionally charged anxious energy. Then when you move on to the other chapters in this book, you'll be more effective in putting together the whole range of anxiety-relief strategies that will work for you.

A "Map" Out of Anxiety

Step 1: Picture Your Anxiety

If you had to draw a picture of your anxiety, what would it look like?

Jason draws his anxiety like this—as a flock of birds he's supposed to be caring for, escaping from their cages into the open sky.

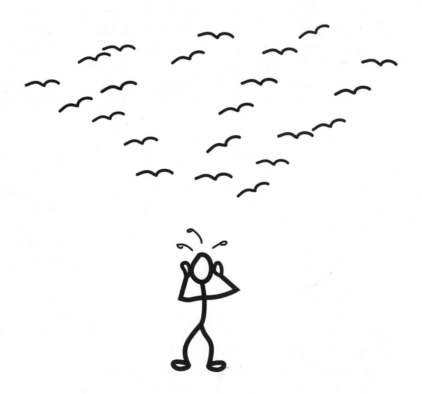

Tina, whose anxiety creeps up on her slowly as she feels herself "sinking under it" or when anxiety is "swirling over her head," draws it this way:

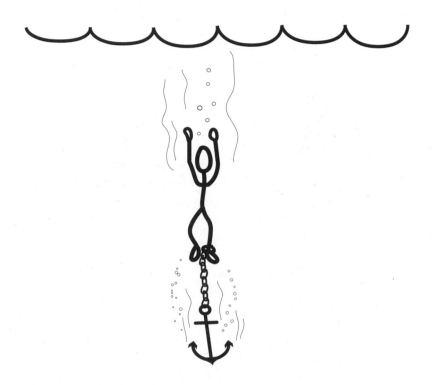

Maxine, who suffers an anxiety disorder, drew her anxiety like a house that's wired with hidden bombs, waiting for her to set them off. That's because she's compelled to check things over and over—like turning off the stove or lights—"because if I don't, the anxiety tells me something bad will happen."

Bill drew his anxiety as an icy blast—freezing the words in his throat...then stiffening all his joints until he's "frozen" with fear.

Why is this step important? Because we can learn to manage anxiety of every kind as we learn how to—

- *recognize its first signs before it takes control of our body, mind, or spirit.*

- *replace its disturbing and uncomfortable sensations—the ones that make us respond in ways we don't like—with a sense of calm.*

- *escape the controlling, life-limiting pressures of anxiety and make choices that allow us to act freely.*

If we want a life of freedom, inner ease, happiness, and productivity, we can have it as we learn how to transform anxious energy into creative energy.

This first step of picturing anxiety begins the necessary work of *creating an objective "distance" between us and our anxious impulses.* Because our anxious impulses feel so automatic, and they seem to be so much a part of us, we need to perform a mental action that is something like an apple peeling itself. We need to create space—a little at first, then more and more as we go—between ourselves and anxious feelings.

This is not at all the same thing as *denying* that you feel anxious. It's not the same thing as *rationalizing* ("It really doesn't affect me *that* much") or *philosophizing* ("What doesn't kill me makes me stronger") or *spiritualizing* ("God must have a good purpose in letting me suffer this way"). Those are excuses for not facing and dealing with anxiety.

"Picturing" anxiety is "peeling the skin off" your anxiety, so you can step back, look at the anxious impulses, and think about them. It will help you gain objective understanding about your anxiety and its triggers. It will help you begin to understand how to respond to anxious impulses calmly and in healthier ways.

How would you picture your anxiety and what it does to you?

Step 2: Name Your Anxiety

Jason named his anxiety the "I fly apart" feeling. "It's like I'm flying into pieces…and I panic, because I feel like I'm going to totally lose control. All my muscles clench, like I'm trying to hold my body together. And if anyone tries to talk to me when I feel like this I'm irritable because I'm so busy trying not to come unglued."

Tina calls her anxiety, the "drowning" feeling. "Life and all these challenges are welling up all around me. Suddenly I feel like I'm in over my head. That's when the panic attacks can come."

Maxine speaks of her "watching for disaster" feeling. "Irrational as it is, it feels like I need to keep checking and checking the stove, the lights, the alarm clock…whatever…or the house will blow up or burst into flames or something. These thoughts crowd out just about every other thought, until I'm driving myself and my family nuts with all this checking."

Maxine says she could also draw another picture of her anxiety and call it the "contaminated house" feeling. She is identifying one of the characteristics of an anxiety disorder, which is that *its triggers can change* or *become multiple triggers.*

"I also have a 'get it off me' feeling. I get anxious when the house feels cluttered or dirty to me. My skin crawls. This can happen even if I've just made everyone scrub and dust every inch of the place. When this feeling comes, I stand in the shower until the hot water runs out, or just wash my hands over and over."

Bill calls his picture of anxiety the "frozen rabbit" feeling. "When anxiety grabs me, I feel like a rabbit that's sensed a hawk circling overhead. The feeling of terror makes me freeze. Physically and mentally I just seize up. I can't work or think. All I can do is shake and hope the threat goes away."

"Naming" your anxiety is another step in placing objective distance between you and the impulse. It also gets you ready for the next important step.

Strategy 3: Feel How Your Body Responds to Anxiety

Jason realized that anxiety creates in him the physical sensation of *weakness* in all his muscles and joints. "I used to say, I feel like I'm losing control, but when I focus in on how my body actually feels I realize that my muscles and joints suddenly get loose and weak."

Tina had a hard time focusing in on her body's response to anxiety. "I've always hated my body because I got the message growing up that I had an unshapely, 'boyish' body. I guess feeling ashamed of my body trained me to live 'apart' from it and not feel what's going on there.

"But when I took the time and concentrated, I realized that anxiety makes my throat get tight and my chest constrict. I guess that's why I feel like I'm drowning. I'm literally not getting oxygen."

Since her "anxiety triggers" change, *Maxine's* body can respond in different ways. "Sometimes it begins with my stomach tightening up. Other times, the nerve endings beneath my skin tingle. Then my muscles tighten because I'm trying not to touch anything."

Bill's response is always the same. "My breathing gets shallow. Sometimes I even hold my breath. All my muscles get rigid, too. I guess I really *become* that 'frozen rabbit' hiding from the predator."

Strategy 3: Recognize the Sources of Your Anxiety

Sometimes our anxiety has one clear, original source. We become anxious because we were once locked in a small space and thought we were going to die in there. But by the time anxiety becomes a life-dominating problem, the anxious impulse has most likely spread from its original trigger into other aspects of our lives. Its influence has *transferred* to triggers that can be totally unrelated to the original trigger.

It's important to identify as many triggers of your anxiety as possible. Here's what you do:

- *Identify when the anxiety first began.* You may need the help of a counselor or therapist to do this. If the anxiety began before you can remember, in early childhood, you may not be able to identify the "historical" first source. If so, don't get hung up on this. What we're doing is "behavioral therapy," not "psychotherapy."

- *Identify as many current anxiety triggers as p⟍* 29
  triggers your anxiety *now?* Even if there are psy⟍
  issues to deal with from the past (and if there a⟍
  chotherapy may be necessary), we can help ourselves gre⟍
  by singling out as clearly as possible the *people, times, objects,*
  or *situations* that trigger anxiety.

- *Pinpoint the ways anxiety "hooks" you.* People, times, objects,
  situations—these create the "setting" in which anxiety comes.
  But the *anxious response* comes from inside you.

This took *Maxine* a good bit of work. She realized that her anxiety disorder has a definite bio-chemical component—but upon
reflection also realized that it had another source. Once the body-
based anxiety began, it also "hooked into" anxieties that had their
source in her spiritual beliefs. A behavior therapist helped her recognize that she carried a deep anxiety that you can commit "the
unpardonable sin." She suffered what's known as "religious scrupulosity," an over-focus on being "imperfect" and "offending God."

Part of Maxine's personal treatment plan included drug therapy,
under the supervision of a psychiatrist. It also required the use of
healthy spiritual practices to counter her spiritually based anxiety
with the help of a spiritual director. (See Chapter 4 on the use of
spiritual practices in relieving anxiety.)

Bill knew immediately that his "frozen rabbit" feeling originated
in early childhood, when one of his parents held the threat of leaving
over the other's head. As all little kids imagine, if you're abandoned
by your parents, terrible things—maybe even death—will "get" you.
Triggered by the anxious thought of being left, Bill's body resisted.
Involuntarily, he held his breath and went into "muscle freeze," in a
survival-instinct attempt to keep the overwhelming terror of aban-
donment from "getting" him.

In adulthood, though, Bill also had a tough time recognizing the
point inside himself where anxiety hooked into him. That's because
he became severely anxious when financial pressures built. He'd
been trained to think that "a real man is successful and doesn't have
financial problems." He was also resistant to getting behavioral help

.d been trained to think, "A man knows how to handle his
⸤oblems." To make things worse, he hated taking medications
.eally needed some biochemical intervention.

Bill benefited from some self-care strategies that helped relieve
mentally based anxiety and some natural supplements. Eventually,
he relaxed enough to accept outside professional help to continue his
healing. (See Chapter 3 for strategies that relieve mentally based
anxiety. Chapter 7 presents a range of natural supplements that
restore inner calm and balance.)

Jason knew immediately most of his anxiety triggers. But a
careful look at every aspect of his life surprised him. He hadn't realized that his diet was creating a problem for him. Adjusting his
eating habits wasn't the easiest thing to do. He liked certain foods
that actually made him feel "keyed up" and lowered his anxiety
threshold. But it was part of the whole-life adjustment Jason was
willing to make. (Chapter 5 describes foods that can create physiological stress and contribute to anxiety.)

How do your anxiety triggers "hook into" you?

Strategy #4: Create a New "Target Feeling"— Calm

Perhaps you've heard that to relieve your anxiety you'll need to
"confront" the things that trigger it. While "exposure therapy" is an
important step, there is another step you need *first*. It's a step that
some behavior therapists skip. But if you learn to do this, you'll find
that you're able to manage anxiety much more quickly.

What we need to know is *how* to create a new "target feeling"—
a relaxed sense of calm, steadiness, peace, and balance. What does it
take for you to experience inner stability?

Anxiety is a very powerful "target feeling." As soon as you
encounter the things that trigger anxiety, your body, mind, and spirit
respond automatically to the threat. This *threat response* becomes
deeply ingrained until our whole being knows how to reproduce
anxiety without any thought at all.

What we need to do is gradually *replace* the threat-response sensations with a different target feeling, or what is known as the *relaxation response.*

The goal is to recondition each aspect of our whole being to produce or "hit" the new target feeling of peace rather than speeding into anxious distress. *The stronger you make your experience of inner calm and stability, the more likely you will be to redirect your focus away from anxious feelings when they arise and, instead, reach the new "target," which is calm stability.*

Chapters 3, 4, and 6 will be especially beneficial in helping you learn a variety of strategies that will produce the "target feeling" of calm and steadiness.

Strategy #5: Touch Base with Your Anxiety Triggers

Exposing yourself to the things that trigger anxiety is the important next step. (You may need the help of a caring professional to do this.)

Here are the elements of exposure therapy:

- *Encounter the object, experience the anxiety.* You'll need to expose yourself to the "forbidden" or "dangerous" thing.

- *"Map" your anxious reaction.* How do you respond physically, mentally, or on a spiritual level? When something triggers anxiety, what is the first feeling you get? Where in your body does anxiety cause a reaction? Does it spread from one part of your body to another? Once anxiety has taken hold, what other aspects of your being does it hook into? Your thoughts? Spiritual beliefs?

- *As your anxiety rises, attempt to create the new target feeling of calm.* This will take practice.

- *Shift your focus to the part of your body that's reacting.* Before your physical reactions take total control, be prepared to take charge of the anxious energy that's running wild in your body.

- *Relax the anxiety out of your body.* If your breathing is affected, use one of the breathing strategies in this book to create a relaxed breathing pattern. If your muscles are tense, use a stretching strategy. If your whole being is coiled like a spring, involve yourself in a more strenuous physical diversion like walking, running, or another form of exercise.

- *Direct the new sense of calm into your thoughts or spiritual awareness.* Speak to your anxious thought-stream or agitated spirit: "Be calm." "Relax…be at peace." "Settle down and feel the calm." Soon you'll find this kind of *over thinking*, which directs your thoughts and soul-stirrings, to be very effective.

What you've done to this point is to take a "short break" from the thing that triggers your anxiety, in order to create a new consciousness inside you while the trigger is present. This may take a few minutes, or, as you become better at it, just a few seconds. In time, it can become automatic. Now…

- *Refocus on the anxiety trigger.* While you are experiencing the new target feeling of calm, examine the person, object, place, or situation that triggered your anxious responses. Take time to dwell on it…as long as you can. The longer you can experience calm in the presence of the trigger, the more you will replace the anxious response with the new *relaxation response.*

- *Practice, practice.* Because anxiety is a powerful sensation, you should practice this type of exposure therapy regularly, until you're quickly able to use this technique anywhere, any time, on your own.

Beyond the Big Picture

Finding relief from life-dominating anxiety involves a bit of work. Now that you have the "big picture," you'll need to fill in the details. Fortunately, the "work" we have to do is wonderful because it involves us in finding a personal self-care strategy that creates calm, stability, and a total approach to restoring well-being.

What mental-anxiety relief strategies will work for you?

Which spiritual practices will relieve the deep-core stresses in your life?

Are there dietary changes you need?

Which natural supplements are effective?

What about physical practices that relieve anxiety?

The chapters that follow will help you create a specific self-care plan personalized to work for you.

3

Mental Anxiety Relief

"Anxiety" is the word we use to describe that emotional cocktail made of one part *fear* and three parts *the sense that something awful and beyond our control* is about to happen. Anxiety is the catch-all term we use when we feel like our world, or some important part of it, is rattling apart. But not all anxiety is the same, so it can't always be treated and relieved in the same way.

As with every health issue, if you treat the symptom and not the root cause, you are never going to cure the real problem.

The fact is, feelings of anxiety can be generated in one of several ways. They can be generated physically, when too many of the "fight or flight" hormones are pumped into our bloodstream. They can be generated by imbalances in our brain chemistry, also when the brain is "mechanically" overwhelmed and struggling to process too much information or conflicting and confusing signals. (See "Bob's Story," on pages 36–37.)

This brings up an important point: When dealing with life-dominating anxiety, it's important to get the help of a professional to determine if our mentally based anxieties are being caused by a physiological problem and, therefore, need to be treated with drug and behavior therapies. While the strategies in this book will benefit even those whose anxiety is generated by brain dysfunctions, pharmaceutical and therapeutic interventions are the most helpful ways of intervening, especially when anxiety is acute and impairs your ability to live well.

Sometimes, too, anxiety is generated by our own minds—that is, *by the way we think*. This would include single thoughts that induce anxiety. ("What if my two-year-old wanders away in this huge crowd?") And it includes patterns of thinking that create anxiety. (We'll look at examples of this later.) We can refer to this as *mentally induced anxiety*, or, simply, *anxious thinking*.

～

BOB'S STORY
When Your Brain Is Shouting for Help

From the time Bob was young, he had a problem with reading. The page would "shimmer" before his eyes. He couldn't retain information. Little wonder then that school work made him anxious, and his grades suffered.

Bob also complained of painful headaches. "It felt like someone had hooked a fish hook through the upper corner of one eye, just a half-inch in from the bridge of my nose. When I'd get a headache—and they were awful headaches, like migraines—it always began in the same spot."

And then there was the anxiety. Bob would become agitated, especially in school when he was supposed to be concentrating. He was diagnosed with an "attention deficit disorder" and placed on Ritalin, which helped him to a small degree. But the headaches and the anxiety did not go away.

Somehow Bob managed to compensate for his reading problem, graduated from college, and stepped into a successful professional career. Biking helped to channel his anxious energies, but the headaches continued. And now, when he read, the vision in one eye would suddenly blank out. Not only that, his lifelong anxiety "spread." Bob was diagnosed with a full-blown anxiety disorder—Obsessive-Compulsive Disorder (OCD).

When Bob's physician took a full medical history, he had a hunch. Bob was sent to an ophthalmologist who understood there is a potential link between visual processing and anxiety.

Tests showed that Bob's eyes were focusing independently of each other. (This accounted for the headaches, because the muscles in his weaker eye were being strained to pull that eye into focus with his dominant eye.) Because he was literally focusing in two different places, his brain was receiving two completely different sets of signals. (This accounted for the sense of anxiety, as his brain signaled it was literally being overwhelmed.) As a result, his brain had developed the habit of shutting out one set of visual signals. (This accounted for the sporadic "blanking out" of vision in Bob's weaker eye.) All these symptoms were the brain's way of shouting for help.

Today, using specially made "prismatic" lenses for reading and work, and using carefully monitored pharmaceuticals, Bob's anxiety has decreased, allowing him to manage his obsessive compulsions.

Our bodies are indeed "fearfully and wonderfully made." They're complex and fascinating. And for that same reason, finding the root cause of an anxiety disorder can be like trying to solve a mystery. Fortunately, Bob's doctor stepped back, looked at all the puzzle pieces of evidence together, and resisted coming to the standard conclusions others had come to. Instead, following a hunch, he sent Bob on to an expert, knowing an expert is someone who can look at symptoms from a new angle, from a viewpoint formed by a different set of skills.

We all need to learn to listen to our bodies and not overlook any of its distress signals. As many specialists know, our bodies are amazingly good at telling us when and where we need help and treatment.

Bottom line: *Be willing to check out any and all possibilities, to see if there is a physiological cause for your anxiety.*

∾

The good news is that we can learn how to recognize and release the crippling inner pressures that anxious thinking produces. In fact, there are simple and effective strategies we can learn, natural therapies we can use to relieve mentally induced anxiety any time, anywhere.

Before we look at these strategies and how to use them, I want to share a word about the ways our minds create mentally induced anxiety.

Anxious Thoughts, Anxious Thought Patterns, and Panic

For many of us, the way our mind works has turned us into "stress batteries." We generate inner pressures and cram all the energy of anxious thinking inside until we're unable to breathe, our body's systems are shutting down, and we're either shaking or numb with fear.

Mentally induced anxiety is generated in one of several ways. Which ones do you recognize?

First, we can have *anxious thoughts*—an over focus and concern on certain issues, events, possessions, or people that are important to us. These can be fairly easy to recognize. Second, we can experience anxiety-producing *thought patterns*—ways we process our thoughts about life that habitually create anxiety. Finally, we can experience *panic attacks* regularly or on occasion, usually because we're subject to circumstances in one part of our life, or in too many aspects of life at once, and they emotionally overwhelm us.

Anxious thoughts can increase the damaging effects of emotionally, spiritually, or physiologically based anxiety by adding more inner pressure to other anxiety-stresses we may already be suffering. For this reason, it's very important for us to recognize the workings of our own mind and learn how to relieve anxious thinking.

Anxious Thoughts

Do any of these examples of anxious thoughts sound familiar to you?

- *I'm tormented with anxiety about my [health, finances, past, future, loved one's safety or well-being, losing something or someone I care about].*

- *I [avoid, freeze up, feel sick, get tearful or angry] when I face personal challenges such as speaking in public, lack of finances or other resources, pressure to perform tasks I'm not good at.*

- *I become anxious about a certain task—such as cleaning, or office paperwork, balancing my checkbook—obsessing until I complete it…or until it's done "right."*

- *I know I am going to [get sick, lose my job, fail, look stupid].*

Anxious thoughts are evidence of an over focus on one fairly clear concern. For instance, we may drive ourselves into an anxious state for days until that messy office is reorganized, but once the last file folder is in place, relief comes and the sick stomach or headache goes. (To return, of course, when the next challenge to our sense of order rises.)

Unpleasant as anxious thoughts are, as soon as the stressor is resolved, the inner discomfort goes immediately. The sun comes out and we can breathe again. Unfortunately, many of us who suffer from anxious thoughts often do little to learn how to manage anxious thinking. We let the tides of life take care of anxiety for us—letting it wash in with one tide of challenging circumstances, and wash out again when we've stressed ourselves by battling anxiously to "set the world right" again. We ignore the high cost to health. We may be programming ourselves for more impairing forms of anxiety—such as panic attacks. And we never learn to manage our "ride" through life.

Life *can* be better. But we need the strategies included in this chapter to smooth the ride and reduce the inner stress of anxiety that is slowly, dangerously, eroding our health and setting us up for serious mental, emotional, and physical illness.

Anxious Thought Patterns

Perhaps you'll also recognize these examples of *anxious thought patterns.*

- *I don't know why, but I have to do things in a certain way, a certain order, or at a certain time, or I get anxious.*

- *Even when nothing is going wrong I think, "Something is always going to go wrong. It's just a matter of what next? And when?"*

- *If I don't [do a certain thing], then [a bad thing] will happen. I won't be able to live with myself if I don't keep [the bad thing] from happening.*

- *Everything is riding on my shoulders. The other people around me are just not good at [doing the all-important task] right. If I leave it to them, it will be a disaster.*

- *I have to solve problems on my own.*

- *I feel uncomfortable expressing my emotions…or even identifying what I'm feeling.*

- *I feel uncomfortable expressing my thoughts, beliefs, or opinions…or have a hard time knowing what it is I do think, believe, or stand for.*

- *I have a hard time focusing on the present moment because I'm caught up in anxious thinking about [past losses] and how I could have prevented them…or about [future goals] and how miserable I'll be if they don't come to fruition.*

Anxious thought patterns can be harder to recognize. They can be so habitual they seem normal to us. And so, like an emotional "weather system," they contribute constant "high pressure" to our inner atmosphere.

Besides making life unpleasant, anxious thoughts and thought patterns can seriously damage our health. According to recent medical studies, stress is a major factor in almost half of the life-threatening illnesses plaguing our culture—from depression and other emotional illnesses to cancer, asthma, osteo- and rheumatoid arthritis, and other diseases of the immune system, and to heart disease, high blood pressure, and chronic headaches and migraines.

Panic Attacks

If you've ever experienced the devastation of a panic attack you never forget it. But do you recognize these conditions that often lead up to an attack?

- *I sometimes find my thoughts or emotions spinning out of control.*

- *I sometimes feel like I'm starting to slide down into a dark tunnel or whirlpool.*

- *Sometimes I feel like I'm being overwhelmed with details and pressures, like the room is filling up with water rising above my head very fast, and I feel pressure in my chest.*

- *Sometimes my heart races for no reason; sometimes I suddenly find it hard to breathe.*

- *Sometimes when I'm inside I suddenly get claustrophobic and have to get outside. Or sometimes when I'm outside I suddenly feel too vulnerable and have to get inside.*

Panic attacks, cardio-respiratory attacks, and phobias can have similar triggers. Those triggers can be biochemical or emotional. When emotional triggers are causing our attacks, they're often linked to past trauma, such as a serious loss, an emotional abuse, a sexual violation, or sometimes to a "wrong" that our sense of ethics tells us we've committed.

What's most difficult about relieving panic attacks that have an emotional trigger is that sometimes the traumatic event doesn't seem like a big issue to us anymore. It's long buried in our past and, we believe, long ago forgotten. We long ago "forgave" the perpetrator. Or we believe we've "grown up" and become a big boy or big girl now and no longer carry the past trauma.

Sometimes, too, we see ourselves as more capable than we are. In fact, super-achievers can and do suffer panic attacks. But because we see ourselves as capable, strong, together, when an attack strikes our first response is to deny we have suffered any trauma or experience fear. ("I'm a Christian, and I forgave the man who sexually assaulted me years ago." "My panic attacks can't be triggered by my personal challenges, I'm the vice president of a company and manage millions of dollars." "I can't be scared about the safety of my child at daycare, I'm a top-ranked female triathlete.")

Most panic attack sufferers rely on anti-panic medications when they feel an attack coming on. These medications quiet, but do not undo, the real fears that often underlie panic attacks—that is, the fear of *being abandoned* or the fear of *being engulfed*. Many panic attack sufferers find great benefit from long-term counseling or therapy. In this way, we can gain a clear understanding of the unconscious emotional habits we formed in response to traumas and overwhelming feelings we experienced before we were mature enough to know how to express them and take charge of our lives again.

"Collateral Discharge"—Negative Emotional Energy Firing into Your Body

How does anxiety exert pressure from our inner being to our physical body? By sending what can be called a "collateral discharge" of negative energy. It's bad enough that anxiety shuts down creative thinking that could help us solve problems as they arise or that it triggers painful emotions. But its inner pressure actually cross-fires tension into our muscles and nerves, slowing our breathing and straining our cardiovascular system. The sudden jolt of pressure triggers the release of hormones needed for "fight or flight," which automatically shuts down the production of hormones needed for healthy metabolism, disease prevention, and cell and tissue repair. Digestion slows or stops cold as blood rushes to your extremities, giving you that cold, sick knot in your stomach.

Given enough anxiety, over enough time, we can truly become "worried sick."

The big question, then, is, How do we relieve the inner pressure caused by *anxious thoughts*, *thought patterns*, and *panic attacks*?

Strategies for Mental Anxiety Relief

Strategy 1: Take the Breath of Life

When anxiety grips us in any form, the first bodily function it clamps down on is our *breathing*. (Next time you're startled or get bad news, notice how automatically you respond by sucking in and holding your breath.) It's as if we're instinctively trying to "freeze" the world that's just spun out of control. In reality, what we're stopping is our normal, healthy, bodily functions. (This works well for rabbits when they're instinctively stilling every muscle and quieting their hearts, trying to be undetectable in the presence of a predator. But it's very unhealthy for human beings.)

The single most important strategy you can use, anywhere at any time, is to restore what I call "the breath of life" to your body. Sometimes this is referred to as "breath work." The beauty of this easy-to-learn strategy is that it offers whole-person benefits—physical, mental, and spiritual—all in one simple package. It shifts your focus off the anxiety-trigger and restores peace and balance to your mind.

Do This

1. **Focus your attention on your breath as you slowly breathe in through your nose. Fill your lungs. Then relax and let the air flood out. Continue.** This strategy shifts your focus off the inner or outer "attacker," and it can bring rapid relief from anxiety. Yes, that other "force" will try to pull your attention back to it. Don't resist or try to "argue" with your anxiety...just keep redirecting your focus back to your breathing. (Anxiety can't be "driven out," but it *can* be ignored until it eases.)

2. **Eventually, move into one of the relaxing breath patterns.** In "breathwork" therapy, certain breathing patterns are known to induce both inner and outer relaxation. Try one of the following (mentally count to the indicated number as you do each breathing segment):

In-breath	Pause	Out-breath	Pause
4	1	8	1
4	1	10	1
6	2	6	2

Note: Your focus is on *developing a steady rhythm* and *slowing* or *balancing your out-breath*. Whenever your focus wanders, and it will, gently turn it back to your breathing.

Strategy 2: Return to Your Senses—Get Grounded

Anxiety *demands* our full attention—mind and body. As anxiety takes hold of our body, we focus on the sensations anxiety produces. We allow our whole flesh-and-blood being with its million miles of nerve endings to become hyper-focused on the physical discomforts of anxiety. Anxiety has invaded our physical being and replaced all other sensations. All we can think of is how bad we feel.

For some of us, the best strategy for escaping anxiety is to redirect our minds to *pleasant physical sensations*. This offers relief by *grounding* our wildly scrambling thoughts and the flailing emotions to objects that feel good and solid to us. Physically, we also evoke a positive response from our limbic system, which will produce a whole-body sense of well-being.

Here are three alternatives.

Do This

1. **Make contact with someone you know who is "in a good place."**

Sometimes contact with a good friend, even via the telephone, will help "ground" us. But it would be far better if we can make real physical contact.

- *Seek the sensation of calm stability you need in the feel of...*
  —a comforting arm around your shoulders

  —a sympathetic hug

  —a neck or shoulder rub

  —an arm in your arm, a hand in your hand

- *"Lean into" the physical sensation*
  —as you relax, focus your attention on the point of contact

  —the calm stability, the strength, or the care of the other person

Experiencing therapeutic touch is a good way to redirect your ~om the swarming anxious thoughts and resulting sensations.

For some of us, an underlying contributor to our anxiety may in fact be that we're suffering from an abysmal lack of caring human contact or a solid sense that someone cares for and about us. Sadly, for many people, this deficit may be a lifelong one. Unfortunately, we've made a cultural joke out of our real human need to be held and touched when our world feels like it's coming apart. "Someone needs a hug" has become a laugh-line. But touch *is* therapeutic. (See the Chapter 6 sidebar on "Healing Touch.")

Don't be hesitant to ask for this kind of help, even from a close friend or family member. The only requirement is that the person you're making contact with be outside and apart from the circumstances that are quaking your world. In this way, they provide the stable ground to counter the drowning swimmer sense anxiety creates in our bodies.

2. Experiment with "scents" that calm you.

Strongly pleasant scents are also effective attention-distracters. They can shift the focus of anxious thinking rapidly, bringing up calming associations and even wonderful memories. The result is to shift us out of mental anxiety and draw us into a more peaceful "head space." Besides providing a mental distraction, pleasing scents can offer physical benefits, too.

Aromas can have a tonic effect on our limbic system. This is where the healing effects of aromatherapy come in. Studies show that one subliminal effect of pleasing scents is that they trigger our body's "deep-relaxation response," which boosts our immune functioning.

You may want to carry with you, in your purse, pocket, or briefcase, one of the aroma therapy oils listed below. These essential oils—and others (feel free to experiment)—can be helpful in redirecting anxious thinking and helping you experience a whole-body relaxation:

chamomile	ginger	rose
clary sage	lavender	sandalwood
geranium	peppermint	wintergreen

GET *HELPFUL* HELP

～

Some people "should" be the ones to support us, naturally speaking. These would include parents, spouses, children, best friends, people in our spiritual community. But very often it's these people who are, ironically, *not* able or willing to do so. It's because they have other agendas to protect, such as their own sense of well-being, or religious beliefs, or *something* else that slips in and takes priority over giving unqualified free support to you.

Yes, this is sad, but it happens all the time. When you're anxious and in need of support...*be wise.*

It does no good to turn to our spouse, parent, friend, child, or church friend for support for the *umpteenth* time...when we've turned to them for support before and come away feeling worse. Trying to make them change into empathetic, supportive people is not your task. Saving your sanity and restoring well-being is.

As the saying goes, "Insanity is doing the same thing over and over, and expecting a different result *this* time." Make sure you get *helpful* help.

Note: You may want to use a diffuser, to "season" the air in your home or office with one of these oils. They can also be used to create a calming bath by adding 2 to 10 drops of oil in warm (not hot) water.

Warning: Keep essential oils away from your eyes and away from small children and pets. Never ingest them.

3. "Ground" yourself.

Some of us "ground" ourselves when anxiety strikes by reconnecting with the physical world in creative ways. Doctors, therapists, and spiritual directors recognize the therapeutic value of literally "mixing it up" with the physical elements.

Even if you have never seen yourself as a "creative type" you may find great release from anxiety and an amazing sense of well-being in turning your mind to…

- *gardening—digging your hands into freshly turned soil*

- *sculpting—reshaping clay*

- *wood- or metalworking—retooling pine or maple…or wrought iron*

- *painting or drawing—capturing the world's blends of color, shape, and texture*

Technically, any action that refocuses our minds away from anxious thinking and physical sensations can act as an agent of calm. (In a later chapter, we'll consider a broader range of physical practices you can add to your self-care strategies.) Redirecting our minds away from anxious thoughts and thought patterns is the main goal. Creative pursuits are helpful in "grounding" us to the calming feel of something solid in our hands.

Strategy 3: Get Out

When anxiety hits, it slowly traps our whole being. We literally zero in on problems. Our eyes focus narrowly and intently. Our mind zooms in on the uncomfortable agitation that's ripping through our nerves and muscles. Our spirit feels like it's been cast into a hellish state. We magnify the anxiety and cause its energy to build, sometimes until the pressure and agitation are physical, mental, and spiritual torture.

Fortunately, there is another simple and important strategy we can use to *get out* of anxiety's tormenting grasp. Learning to shift our focus from narrow to broad can quickly dispel anxious thoughts and feelings, and its a practice that's easy to master.

Narrow focus is what we do when we're intent on some urgent activity. For example, in looking for a dropped contact lens, your mind, eyes, and your whole physical being (and maybe your emotions, too) zero in. Narrow focus increases tension throughout our whole being and makes small matters become intensified and loom large.

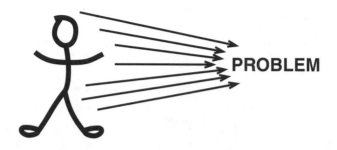

Narrow Focus

When you find the contact lens, you relax, breathe, and return to the wider avenues of living you were on before you lost the lens. Suddenly the (literally) bigger and more important things in your life come back into focus.

Broad focus is what we do when we're daydreaming, letting our eyes relax and wander "wherever." We stare vacantly at distant hills, the drifting clouds, or some corner of the ceiling...not so much seeing with our eyes as "envisioning" our life from a sort of "pinnacle of emotional and spiritual awareness"...a clearer, calmer vantage point. Our whole being relaxes. We experience physical calm. We gain emotional perspective. We may even sense our spirit is suddenly more in tune with God. In short, we've moved ourselves *out* of the state where mental anxiety occurs.

Broad Focus

How do we learn the strategy of shifting from *narrow* to *broad focus?*

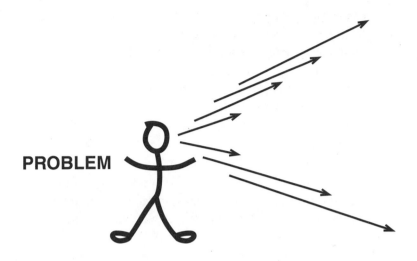

Do This

1. Make time to get outdoors for a walk. When this isn't possible, take a comfortable seat near a window. (You may want to use Strategy 1, *Breathing,* to help you get relaxed.)

2. Let your eyes focus on distance...and relax. "Focus" isn't exactly what we're about. We're opening our peripheral vision.

3. When intrusive thoughts come...gently turn your mind back to broad focus. If necessary, use a *focus word* or *focus thought.*
Sometimes it's helpful to have a single word that keeps us focused on what we're doing. It's so easy for anxious thoughts to keep whispering...or shouting...at us. It's a mistake to try to fight these thoughts, because we wind up engaging with them, waging a tension-filled battle within our own being. But a single, simple, *focus word* or *focus thought* can be helpful in returning your mind to what it was doing—relaxing—when anxious thoughts tried to take it captive again.
You may prefer to find a specific passage from the scriptures as your focus. The Bible is full of wonderful promises—of peace, stability, and well-being. As you read the scriptures, write out one or

more of the passages that speak to your inner being on a small note card. Keep that card with you in your wallet, purse, or briefcase.

Or you may want to choose an *image* from Scripture. Images are like wordless messages from God. They speak to the deepest levels of our being, which is why some of the most powerful passages in the Bible are stories and parables.

Personally, my favorite image from the scriptures is that of the "River of God." Not only does this image "run" throughout the whole Bible, from Genesis to Revelation (a fact I find intriguing in itself), it plants in my spirit a beautiful representation of the Spirit of God, continually encircling the earth with life-restoring energy... as one passage puts it, a divine power and will that is for the healing of people of all nations.

Meditating on this rich image of the powerful, unstoppable flow of divine healing energy creates an amazing peace and positive atmosphere in my soul and provides relief from spiritually based anxieties.

4. "Hold" this state of open, relaxed consciousness. Give your body and spirit time to relax into the calm state of being your mind has opened up.

Strategy 4: Scan Your Mind for "Bad Weather" Patterns

Some of our anxiety, as we've seen, comes from *patterns* in our thinking. Some of these patterns have been part of us so long they're now invisible to us. And yet their powerful effect on us is much like the huge bad weather patterns centered hundreds of miles away, causing storm-fronts to blow through our neighborhood.

Once we've discovered how to create a safe zone of *calm awareness* by learning how to get out and away from anxiety, we can take more steps in learning how to manage mentally based anxiety. This may include learning how to become aware of these deep-pattern mental habits that cause us distress.

"Scanning" our own thought patterns is, to use the weather metaphor again, like employing Doppler radar to detect atmospheric disturbances. The atmosphere we're scanning, however, is our own mental climate. How does this work?

Do This

1. Set aside time each day to "scan" the content of your thoughts. You may wish to journal, so you can track your inner climate patterns over time in order to see how dominant they are. Become aware of patterns such as:

- *Perfectionistic or idealistic thinking*—Sometimes there is a huge gap between the high standards we hold and reality. Our anxiety results from the inner tension we feel between the way we *think* the world should be and the way it is. Perfectly put-together people…and also people full of bright, shining ideals…can suffer enormous anxiety.

- *Critical or judgmental thinking*—On the flip side, anxiety can come from holding standards that are hard or harsh. The evidences are sarcasm, caustic comments, put-downs. Proclaiming who's going to heaven and who's not. Again, anxiety can come from knowing down deep that few people meet our standards—not even us.

- *Self-negating thinking*—"What I want doesn't really matter." "What I feel or think isn't important." "What's important is what my [spouse, children, parents, God] wants." The truth is, what we think and what we want *always* counts. It always needs to be figured into the mix. When we have disregarded our own thoughts and feelings long enough, the tension (also sadness and anger) we've been ignoring *will* work its way out…in anxiety.

- *Self-destructive thinking*—One workshop attendee said, "One day I realized I'd been telling myself how much I'd hated my life for years…and that every morning for a month I'd been waking up thinking about how to commit suicide." Self-destructive thinking need not be as acute as this man's to become a major trigger of anxiety. "I hate my [body, face, hair, hips, laugh, stupid brain]" has the potential to produce anxiety because they increase tension between you and *you*.

- *Blame, powerlessness, and "victim" thinking*—When our thoughts center around the way "other people" or "life" continually wounds us, we have given away our personal power to make positive changes and move on with life. Anxiety can spring from the resulting tension.

- *"What if? thinking*—Some of us are stuck in the game of "What if?" "What if I do *this*…and something horrible happens?" The good news is that game works two ways. Playing "What if I do *this*…and something *good* happens?" is the direction we need to head.

- *Obsessive and intrusive thinking*—Generalized anxiety crosses a line and takes on the force of an anxiety disorder when thoughts become obsessive and intrusive. These are thoughts that literally push out the work or play your mind *would* be thinking about…except that these thoughts are forcefully commanding your attention so that it's impossible to focus on the activities you'd rather be doing.

2. Do whatever needs to be done to repattern your thought patterns.

- We all need help, from outside voices, to reexamine thoughts that have power over us. In the case of common anxiety, a wise friend, counselor, or member of the clergy can help point out your negative thought patterns and help you focus on more positive thoughts. When anxiety is acute, chronic, or life-dominating, professional help is needed.

- Learn how to "rescript" your thinking. Every time an anxiety-producing thought pattern moves in, we can counter it with strong, positive, calming thoughts.

Anxious Script: "Having this chronic illness means the life I've loved is at an end."

Calm Script: "I'm going to search for alternative treatments. And I'm going to focus on doing as much as I'm able to, because I want the quality of my life to remain high."

Anxious Script: "If…[he/she]…[leaves me, dies] …I won't be able to face life."

Calm Script: "It will really hurt, but I *will survive.* Everyone goes through serious losses in life, and I know I can figure out how to overcome that hurt, too."

Anxious Script: "What if I try to change jobs/ move/get out of this bad relationship, and the worst happens?"

Calm Script: "What if I make the change I need to make…and go through the work and turmoil change always brings…and find out my life can be as great as I'd like it to be?"

Anxious Script: "I need to [check something, touch/don't touch an object, repeat this thought] or something terrible will happen."

Calm Script: "Nothing bad is going to happen. It's the compulsion talking. I can stop repeating this behavior and things will actually be fine."

Every time we replace an anxiety-producing thought with calming thoughts, we are repatterning the way we think and winning the battle.

Strategy 5: "Face Down" the Fear

Anxiety is the sign that our "fight or flight" instinct is working. Whatever the perceived threat may be, our whole being is tuned for an attack. The first three strategies will help you create a safe, calm mindset...a sort of mental place "above and apart from" the anxiety. The fourth strategy will help you learn to calmly and objectively observe the workings of your own mind and learn to work with your own anxious thoughts.

People who become overwhelmed by anxiety that will not give way to these simpler strategies—and this includes those of us dealing with anxiety disorders—will eventually need to *face the fear* that's undermining our peace and stability. We will need to expose ourselves to the thoughts, persons, places, objects, or activities that trigger anxious behaviors.

Do This

1. **Talk to a "safe" person about your anxiety.** Every kind of anxiety makes us feel vulnerable. A measure of healing comes from telling someone who is trustworthy and confidential what our anxiety is about. General anxiety may lose its hold as we talk to close friends or family members (but *never* to young and dependent children). Life-dominating anxiety requires us to seek help from caring professionals.

"Safe" people act as surrogates when we need to download our anxiety. They allow us to face our *feelings* about the person, place, or thing that's triggering anxiety *before* facing the anxiety trigger itself. They help us sort out our fears and plan strategy.

2. **Plan your strategy.** Sometimes people in our lives keep things upset and in turmoil to control us in some way. A counselor will help us spot these people, figure out what they're up to, and discern how the anxiety they produce in us keeps us under their thumb. Counselors will also help us plan a strategy that will help us stop playing into their hands.

Sometimes we may need to expose ourselves to the place, activity, or object that triggers anxiety. A counselor will help us learn how to safely expose ourselves to the fear or perceived danger in a way that is helpful and healing—not destructive.

3. Create a program that will bring you into contact with the anxiety trigger regularly. At first, you may be able to handle exposure to your anxiety trigger *one time*. That is a victory. Claim it. It may be a month, a week, or day before you can repeat that victory…but creating a plan that brings you into regular contact with the anxiety trigger is important.

Just as your anxious response has worn a path in your mind… you can create a new path in your mind that meets the anxiety producer in a new and different way, with calm stability and confidence.

Deeper Still

Our mind is one aspect of our inner being. Our spirit is another. Spiritually based anxiety can be as crippling as any other form. In the next chapter, we'll look at strategies for releasing anxiety generating from this deepest part of ourselves.

4

Spiritually Based Anxiety Relief

*I*n the Hebrew scriptures the psalmist shouts out, in a state of anxiety that has pushed him near to despair: "From the depths I cry out..." He is crying for relief because, on top of all the other agonies in his life, his spirit feels abandoned. He believes he's been cut off from divine help, and that he's been left forever alone. He's expressing terrible anxiety, and you get the sense that the feelings are welling out, not from his head but from the core of his being...somewhere deep in his chest or gut.

Those of us who have suffered from anxiety or anxiety disorders know that when anxiety has us in its grasp we really do feel, down in a core place in our being, that we're being crushed or we're coming apart. If anxiety is intense enough, we may feel that our essential "spark" of life is going out and we're dying.

The Spirit Connection

The medical community has recently acknowledged the power of the mind–body connection in healing. What many healthcare professionals are less comfortable talking about is the mind-body-*spirit* connection and the role our spirit plays in our health and well-being. Perhaps this is because the existence of the human spirit is not provable scientifically.

People of various religious backgrounds define "spirit" differently. For our purposes, let's define *spirit* as the seat of our innermost drives. Spirit is the life-energy that comes from our desire to live, love, and act according to our most important values. It constantly energizes our thoughts, emotions, and actions. When we're headed in, say, a career direction that's wrong for us, the deep discomfort we feel—sometimes long before our heads catch on—is our spirit telling us we're off the life-path we need to be on.

Our spirit is also the aspect of ourselves that is acutely aware of our relationship to our ultimate values, and so it affects how we feel in what we might call "life-source relationships"—in relation to ourselves, to significant others, and to God. When we've gone against a value—one of those inner laws we live by—the distress we feel is our spirit telling us we've violated one of those rules and done damage to one or more of those important relationships.

When our deepest desires are crushed, when something we've done has weakened or severed a life-source relationship, our spirit can *feel* "cut off" from everyone and all that we hold dear and important—maybe even cut off from divine help. This is *spiritually based anxiety*.

Because the three aspects of our whole being—body, mind, and spirit—are interrelated, anxiety that's generated in our inmost being will affect our physical and mental well-being.

Unfortunately, many of us are successful at ignoring signals from our spirit. The outer world, with its constant demands, grabs most of our attention, time, and energy. Very few of us develop the skill of personal reflection or self-examination that leads to a greater, deeper self-awareness.

Fear is also a factor. It's terrifying to face reality when we feel separated from, or in danger of losing, our connection to an inner-lifesource when we sense it's necessary to our survival. For these reasons, spiritually based anxiety is a bit harder to detect than anxiety from other sources.

Nonetheless, when our spirit is in trouble it constantly sends out signals. We can read these signals as they show up in different forms of distress in the various aspects of our being—body, mind, or emotions. Consider these examples.

John, Debra, and Phoebe

John's first marriage ended in divorce when he left his wife and young son for Claire. Even though John and Claire's newborn girl is in good health, John has been gripped by nighttime panic attacks, centered around unreasonable fears that the baby will die. In conversation with his clergyman he admits he has never dealt with guilt about his first marriage and leaving his young son.

Debra, a successful physician, had a dad who was one of those wonder-fathers. There for her every step of the way, cheering her on, encouraging her…all the way through college and med school. She was obviously the brightest sun in his sky…and he was hers. Now he has terminal stomach cancer. Debra is suffering from an anxiety so powerful her hands shake. Suddenly, for the first time in her self-assured life, she is second-guessing her diagnosis and fearful about the treatment plans she's writing. She cannot think clearly… and rocks between despair, numbness, and deep rage…especially at God, for "letting this happen" to her father.

Phoebe is a classic burden-bearer. Along with running a household and a struggling, small business, she is taking care of a chronically sick child and an ailing in-law. At work, at home, in her community service group, she is everyone's "go to" girl, "therapist" and "surrogate mom"—the source of well-being for literally dozens of people. Even though nightmares about drowning began shaking her awake in cold sweats, Phoebe just kept charging ahead. And on days when her stomach was in knots, she popped antacids and plowed on. "Sure I have anxieties," she admits. "Lots of them. But I can't afford a shrink…or even to take a day off." But then burning in her joints and other devastating physical symptoms led to the diagnosis of fibromyalgia, an illness that could be psychosomatically induced.

We need to recognize when anxiety is originating in the deep core of our being. And then we need to learn how we can free ourselves from its devastating effects.

∿

BEWARE OF SPIRITUAL PEOPLE WHO "PRACTICE MEDICINE" WITHOUT A LICENSE

• Jonathan and Terri's 9-year-old son, Daniel, had Obsessive-Compulsive Disorder. Their pastor felt he had a demon. Jonathan was told, "You must have done something to allow Satan to have access to your son."

• Leslie suffered from rheumatoid arthritis. When she asked the elders of her church to pray for her, they confronted her. "You must have sin in your life. And your sickness is God's way of warning you to stop whatever secret sin you're involved in."

• Dale's best friend insisted her panic attacks would stop if she prayed a certain prayer a certain way. When that didn't work, her friend insisted she see a traveling faith healer who was coming to her church. When that didn't work, her friend returned this diagnosis: "You're not serving God with your life. You're living totally for yourself and your own happiness. I think the truth is you're not saved, and you're going to hell. Your spirit is telling you to repent."

• Jake's church was helping him through a time when his anxiety disorder prevented him from working. One day his pastor phoned to say Jake ought to be giving more to the church. "After all, if you don't give back to God he might remove his hand of blessing. Your troubles are bad now, but if you cheat God of his due, things could get worse."

Hard to believe such monstrous and ignorant statements are being made by "spiritual" people? This brand of spiritual abuse—what I call "diagnosing and prescribing without a license"—happens all the time. The very people who are supposed to be the embodiment of light, grace, and compassion are full of darkness, legalism, and judgment.

Fortunately, the specific people mentioned found other spiritual communities to support them. And they found doctors who detected the *physiological*, not spiritual, bases for their symptoms.

Anxiety is not necessarily "evidence" of a spiritual problem. When your spiritual community is harming you and not helping you...move on. Find one that is compassionate and realistic about the needs of the human body, the mind, and the spirit.

As someone very famous once said, no one can thrive in a spiritual atmosphere that "binds heavy burdens on people's backs" (see Matthew 23:4).

∽

What's Ripping You Apart Inside?

Spiritually based anxiety is generally caused by the fact that two inner forces are in opposition. We feel like we're being "torn apart."

Picture yourself holding onto the engine of a train with one hand and the first boxcar with the other hand. As the engine begins to pull in one direction down the tracks, *you* are the coupling that's bearing all the tension. You *have* to go where this engine is headed. But the boxcar won't budge. And inside that boxcar is a treasure that's of incredible value to you. Someone precious; something dear. Some goal you can't live without achieving. Without it, you don't see how you can even go on living.

And there you are, straining between the unstoppable and powerful force of life as it moves ahead...and the thing you dare not let go of because you'll suffer unbearable anguish without it. It's no wonder we can feel fear and even terror, as if life itself is ending.

If these were real cars on a real train, your muscles would tremble and shake, and eventually you'd have to let go. But these are spiritual forces inside you, and you're left with a spirit that's trembling and weak because it's stuck in ripped-apart mode. And here's another thing: Sometimes it's very hard to see what's inside that boxcar we're trying not to let go of. It can be some treasure we seized—because we sensed it gave life and meaning and joy to us long ago, and we no longer see how vital, how essential, it is to our existence.

That is a picture of spiritual-based anxiety: the power of it, the fact that it's about things that are fundamentally important to us, and how we can *still* be utterly blind to the conflict that's pulling our spirit in opposing directions, which causes anxiety.

The following is a brief list of spiritual conflicts that may be causing you anxiety. Which ones can you identify in yourself? To better assess your range of needs, try to rate their intensity. Read the following statements, and check the degree to which you sense the strain of these inner tensions.

Anxieties About Myself

- I cannot forgive myself for something awful I did...or something important I failed to do.

    ____ *Never*____ *Sometimes*____ *Often*____ *Daily*____ *Obsessively*

- I cannot get myself to do something important, something I believe I *should* be doing.

    ____ *Never*____ *Sometimes*____ *Often*____ *Daily*____ *Obsessively*

- I say I believe or want one thing, but often do something quite the opposite.

    ____ *Never*____ *Sometimes*____ *Often*____ *Daily*____ *Obsessively*

- I am not the husband/wife...parent/child...successful person...spiritual person...I believe I should be.

    ____ *Never*____ *Sometimes*____ *Often*____ *Daily*____ *Obsessively*

- I hate, dislike, distrust, or disgust myself. I hate, or dislike my appearance, personality, or some characteristic about me.

    ____ *Never*____ *Sometimes*____ *Often*____ *Daily*____ *Obsessively*

Anxieties About My Life Circumstances

• I am afraid of losing something—my *job* and the security it gives, a *possession* or *pastime* that gives me joy, a *position* that gives me meaning or status, or my *health*.

_____ Never_____ Sometimes_____ Often_____ Daily_____ Obsessively

• I am not on the life path I want to be on. I honestly wish I was doing something else with my life.

_____ Never_____ Sometimes_____ Often_____ Daily_____ Obsessively

• I am not living where I want to live. I honestly wish I was living somewhere else.

_____ Never_____ Sometimes_____ Often_____ Daily_____ Obsessively

• I am at odds with the group of people I'm involved with—at work, in my general or spiritual community. I honestly wish I had a different set of peers.

_____ Never_____ Sometimes_____ Often_____ Daily_____ Obsessively

Anxieties in My Relationships with Other People

• I fear that someone important to me is going to stop liking me, favoring me, or that he or she will leave me.

_____ Never_____ Sometimes_____ Often_____ Daily_____ Obsessively

• I fear that someone important to me is trying to force me to do things his or her way, maybe even trying to take over and dominate my life.

_____ Never_____ Sometimes_____ Often_____ Daily_____ Obsessively

• I feel as if someone is violating my will or my right to be an individual.

_____ Never_____ Sometimes_____ Often_____ Daily_____ Obsessively

• I feel as if I must get someone to do something, or believe something, or bad things will happen to them.

_____ *Never*_____ *Sometimes*_____ *Often*_____ *Daily*_____ *Obsessively*

• Someone is abusing me in one or more of the following ways: physically, mentally, emotionally, spiritually.

_____ *Never*_____ *Sometimes*_____ *Often*_____ *Daily*_____ *Obsessively*

• I know something bad is happening to another person, and I am not speaking up or doing anything to prevent it.

_____ *Never*_____ *Sometimes*_____ *Often*_____ *Daily*_____ *Obsessively*

• I am angry at someone, but I'm afraid or unwilling to confront them or resolve the issue.

_____ *Never*_____ *Sometimes*_____ *Often*_____ *Daily*_____ *Obsessively*

Anxieties in My Relationship with God

• I live with the fear that I'm really on my own in this life—that something terrible can happen and no one, not even God, will come to my assistance.

_____ *Never*_____ *Sometimes*_____ *Often*_____ *Daily*_____ *Obsessively*

• I believe I've let God down, or made God very unhappy with me.

_____ *Never*_____ *Sometimes*_____ *Often*_____ *Daily*_____ *Obsessively*

• I believe God is angry at me, or wants to punish me for doing something wrong.

_____ *Never*_____ *Sometimes*_____ *Often*_____ *Daily*_____ *Obsessively*

• I believe that God is going to allow something bad to happen to me to "wake me up" or "teach me a lesson."

_____ *Never*_____ *Sometimes*_____ *Often*_____ *Daily*_____ *Obsessively*

• I am deeply angry, sad, or disappointed with God for allowing something bad to happen to me. I still believe in God…I just don't understand God or know how to trust Him any more.

_____ *Never*_____ *Sometimes*_____ *Often*_____ *Daily*_____ *Obsessively*

If you answered "daily" or "obsessively" to some of these questions, you should consider contacting a healthcare professional as you practice the strategies outlined in this book. And even if you answered "sometimes" or "often," you should consider making time daily for the spiritual self-care practices I've outlined.

When we begin to recognize the inner forces that are in opposition, we need a plan of action. By learning how to resolve conflicts of the spirit we relieve the deep tension that's pulling us apart.

Strategies for Relieving Spiritually Based Anxiety

Strategy 1: Praying "In-Flow"

Many of us find ourselves caught in a spiritual bind when anxiety hits. Prayer is the means of connecting with God, whom we recognize as the source of our life and ultimate well-being, but sometimes it's difficult to pray. We can experience conflict in our spirit for one of several reasons:

• We've never thought of turning to God, because we're pragmatic, self-reliant, independent.

℞

RELIGIOUS ANXIETIES AND OBSESSIONS

∼

Sometimes spiritual people suffer anxiety over whether or not they're making God unhappy or angry. This can be a factor in common anxiety if you're a devout person. It can also be a factor in an anxiety disorder. In the latter case, you can feel acute anxiety, thinking that God is watching you intently, picking apart every thought, action, word, and desire. In its acute form, your anxiety can tell you you're on your way to damnation…or already suffering the pains of hell.

Religious *scrupulosity*, as it's known, requires outside intervention. This can come from a general counselor or therapist, or a wise spiritual director or counselor—as long as the individual can help you keep your faith intact while he or she is helping you recognize the unbalanced thinking that's causing you to suffer.

If your anxiety comes from *scrupulosity,* it will be important for you to learn how to separate good *spiritual convictions* or *values* from the unhealthy *voice of criticism, judgment,* and *condemnation*. A wise, caring professional will help you with your thought process by helping you:

- Recognize the "voice" that says your every move is offensive or sinful.

- Challenge the anxiety you feel by testing the offensive thought, desire, or action to see that the God of life does not abandon or condemn you on your human journey.

- Help you rethink your spiritual convictions, keeping intact what's good and healthy about them and letting go of what's unhealthy, anxiety-producing, and destructive.

If scrupulosity is part of an Obsessive-Compulsive Disorder, you can also benefit from one of several antianxiety medications, none of which will cause you to lose your faith. Instead, they will cause your faith to go through a wonderful revolution, landing you in a good place with yourself, others, and with God.

The fact is, ridding yourself of scrupulosity will free you to find the settled peace that is one of the wonderful signs of a healthy, maturing, spiritual life.

- We've been taught that telling God we're anxious is a sign that we don't trust, and that's evidence we don't have faith. God only answers our prayers when we "have faith."

- We've been taught that venting anger (which can accompany anxiety) at God is "a sin." God, who is holy and deserves only reverence and respect, will be displeased.

- We've been taught only rote prayers, or "formula" prayers, that will get God to respond in the way we want.

After living my whole life in and around various spiritual communities of devout people, I believe a word about prayer is in order. When it comes to the way we pray, so many of our religious attitudes create pathologies and dysfunctions. We may indeed be people of faith, but we can also have many unhealthy views of God, along with unhealthy views of ourselves in relation to God.

Many of us pray the way we feed the right combination of coins into a vending machine—expecting the right product to drop out the chute. But God is not a vending machine, and prayer is not about being in control. It's not using the right combination of words so that God will give us what we want. Many of us were taught that honesty, including anxiety, anger, or sadness, were not the right coins to drop into God's slot.

Some of us also pray as if God is utterly fragile and easily offended, almost as if God will be horrified and flee the room unless we speak nicely and well, and have impeccable etiquette. One "bad" word or an "irreverent attitude" and God will scream or faint or punish us. But God is not Miss Manners, and He is not thrown into a holy tizzy by our gut-honesty or by the vocabulary we use when we're in distress.

Some people have been taught to believe that having faith means passively waiting for God to act. But many of us have learned that when we add together self-determined effort *plus* faith amazing things happen. Maybe this is because it's easier to steer a ship that's in motion than one that's in dry dock.

Learning to pray "in flow" is one important strategy that can relieve spiritually based anxiety.

Do This

If your anxiety is at peak...

1. Get alone...and vent. Being by yourself is important because you're going to be less likely to censor your feelings, thoughts, and words. When you are alone...without polite preliminaries, and without censoring...let the words flow. Even if emotional intensity builds, keep the words coming until you feel the energy abate.

At other times...

1. Get alone, get quiet, and breathe. Setting aside time and a place to pray is something few of us do. Maybe it's because we only think of praying as "an obligation," or we only pray when we're in need. Praying "in flow" is important to maintaining good health.

2. "Check in" with your spirit to see if you're feeling in conflict. Some of us pray "from our heads," that is, we say what we *think* we should say. But God already knows what we're thinking and feeling. We're the ones more likely to be out-of-touch by ignoring unpleasant conflicts—especially if they make us feel bad about ourselves. No one wants to see themselves in a negative light.

3. Describe the feeling; if necessary, give it a name. Anxiety may make you feel *frozen* inside, unable to think or decide anything. Or you may feel like the floor has dropped open and you feel *unsteady, ungrounded,* or like you're *falling.*

4. Blame whoever you need to blame for your distress. What? Yes, let the blame fly. While 90 percent of our blaming is misplaced, it's human to feel that someone is always responsible for unpleasant situations. We try to attach our bad feelings to someone or something, and when there's no one else, we blame God. Venting blame gets it out of the way. This is important if praying in-flow is going to have healing value...so let it rip...until you feel the angry or sad *energy* of blame abate.

5. Say what you're going to *do* now. When the emotional intensity is gone, when we're through blaming, now we can face the truth.

Probably no one is to blame. In any case, *we* are the only ones who have the power *to take the next, real-life, positive step.* Out loud, go through all your options, however small or big they might be. Commit yourself to taking the next step that seems right to you. Ask God to show you the next step. Try several options to see which one works best. Good spiritual health includes getting out of "stuck mode" and beginning to move ahead.

   6. Ask for strength and direction. While you're keeping one eye on the road ahead, commit yourself to keeping the other one peeled for outside help and guiding signs. Because God is not limited, strength and direction can come to us from anywhere. And when we're more relaxed and open we're amazed to find that it does.

   When we've cleared our spirit of anxiety—along with clouding emotions and blame—we really can sense ourselves reconnecting with divine strength and direction again.

   It took a lot of coaching for Phoebe, "everybody's everything," to give herself permission to pray "in flow." "What if I blurt out something that sounds just awful—even sort of blasphemous—and make God angry?" she balked. The question was *not* how angry would she make God. The question was, how secretly angry at God *was* she?

   When she finally let herself go, no blasphemous words came out—just the terror she'd carried all her life. Phoebe had been severely and chronically neglected as a little girl, and down deep she believed that when she needs help most *no one* would be there to help her. This fear of abandonment-to-the-worst was at the root of her beliefs. But she recognized this only when she heard the words flow out from this deep place of fear, "*I'm* the one who has to be there to help everyone, because *you're* never there when anyone needs you." It actually shocked her to say out loud what she really thought about God.

   That's when Phoebe realized she'd been carrying the weight of her personal world on her own shoulders. At a deep level, she believed that when things went wrong God would not be there to help. The resulting stress had spiritually, emotionally, and physically worn her out and made her ill. Phoebe benefited further by trying

Strategy 4, (p. 75), allowing her concept of God to have a "make-over."

Strategy 2: Have a Spiritual Confidant

Confession, as the saying goes, is good for the soul. Sadly, not many of us have someone we feel safe bearing our souls to. By safe I mean *able to talk about whatever we think, feel, or believe without fear of being rejected, shamed, made to feel more guilty than we already feel, or seeing shock or dismay in the other person's eyes.* I don't mean someone to "read us the riot act" about our wrong-doing, lack of faith, or sinful behavior."

Soul care, to begin with, needs to be more like going to a hospital emergency room. When you're bleeding from the neck or doubled over in pain, no one in the E.R. begins treating you by trying to find out "what you did wrong" that got you in this condition even if you really did do something boneheaded and injured yourself. In fact, soul care is even trickier than physical care, and it requires wisdom and grace. That's because in the face of blame and criticism, we all retreat and hide, pretending we're okay even when we're not. (Who needs to add the weight of guilt and shame on top of anxiety? As Bugs Bunny's feathered friend, Daffy, says in the cartoons, "Not *this* little black duck.")

We need spiritual confidants who are full of grace—at least that. If we're fortunate, also a bit of wisdom. Having one person on the planet to whom we can open our souls is an important strategy for relieving spiritually based anxiety. In the presence of grace, wisdom, and nonanxious acceptance of who we are, oddly enough we're able to get around to admitting the wrongs we've done and the good we've failed to do.

Do This

1. Find a spiritual counselor or spiritual director with whom you can meet on a regular basis—someone with whom you can be absolutely free, open, and honest.

This may not be a church official. Not everyone is gifted in the soul care department. Find someone who is:

- *Relaxed and strong.* When we experience anxiety, we need someone to be calm and provide solidity.

- *Without a personal agenda.* When we feel someone is trying to convert us to a religion, belief, opinion, course of action, or cause—or when someone "needs to be needed"—that's a sign they're putting their own agenda before your need. A spiritual confidant is there for *you.*

- *Both spiritual and pragmatic in their approach to life.* You need someone who supports your spiritual values, and is, at the same time, practical. Our spiritual convictions need grounding in everyday reality.

- *Confidential. (Period.)*

- *Willing to let us own our emotions, thoughts, and decisions.* If a spiritual confidant tells you, "You shouldn't feel...or think...that way" run. Separating us from our thoughts, emotions, and our physical feelings is the route to infirmity in mind, body, and spirit.

- *Willing to let us have our own journey and learn for ourselves.* A wise spiritual confidant will be willing to let us ask questions, explore, and learn on our own. They may speak from their perspective, but allow us to have our own experiences.

- *Strong enough to intervene when we're in danger.* If we are endangering our health and well-being, we need someone who will take appropriate steps to get us the help we need. (We should agree with a spiritual confidant up front when they can suspend confidentiality if that becomes necessary.)

- *Sets appropriate boundaries.* A spiritual confidant is not a surrogate spouse or parent. A spiritual confidant keeps clear lines between a physical or romantic relationship and the support they're offering. If these lines begin to blur for you, or you sense them blurring for the other person, you should acknowledge the change. It may be necessary to move on to someone else.

2. Meet on a regular basis. Monthly or quarterly may be often enough. Weekly, or even more frequently may be necessary. *Regularly* is the important part. Make emergency contact when necessary. Be sure you can communicate with your spiritual confidant as needed.

3. Be as candid and confessional as you can be. This means making mostly "I" statements. "I think…" "I feel…" "I did [or didn't do]…" "I believe [or don't believe]…"

4. Be candid about your belief system. Often, spiritually based anxiety is based in a belief system that could benefit by being examined, challenged, or developed. Together, explore your answers to questions such as:

- What standards do you judge yourself by?

- What standards do you believe God judges you by?

- What do you believe God's obligation is when it comes to caring for you and your safety and well-being?

5. Be open to challenge; be open to exploring new views. Sometimes we are our own worst enemies, and do things that cause ourselves trouble, stress, and anxiety. Be open to examining the things you do…or fail to do…that generate anxiety. At a deeper level, sometimes our beliefs need reexamination. Be open to direction and dialogue, when your actions (or inactions) or your beliefs are the source of your anxiety. (See Strategy 4, p. 75.)

Good soul care, with the help of a spiritual confidant, goes a long way toward dealing with the energy of anxiety.

John, who was mentioned earlier, benefited greatly from working with a spiritual confidant—in his case, a spiritual director he met through his church. He was able to sort out the conflicts created in his spirit when he walked out on his first wife and child for someone new. This included facing the real guilt he carried over leaving them, which caused hurt and anguish especially to his young son. He also had to deal with the anxiety aroused because of the mistaken image of God he carried—of a vindictive God who would punish him in the most hurtful way possible by taking his newborn daughter's life.

Strategy 3: Build an Inner Sanctuary of Calm

Many of us don't like to be alone and quiet. We feel like we need background noise and activity. Often that's because when we're alone and quiet we become anxious. We "feel uneasy." Or our inner climate may be full of uncomfortable feelings, such as regret, unforgiveness, bitterness toward ourselves and others, fear, grief, or anger. So we avoid going alone into our own soul.

Strategies 1 and 2 are "inner housekeeping" plans. They help us clean "clutter and debris" out of our soul. Learning how to visit the sanctuary of inner calm we're creating is the next step in relieving spiritually based anxiety. Just as athletes do crunches, leg-lifts, and torso twists to build physical "core strength," we can use this strategy to build a spiritual core of strength—that is, a deep state of peace.

Do This

1. **Locate a quiet spot, where you can be alone.** I recommend you find several spots actually, because, on a given day, one may be invaded or inaccessible. Inside, you may want to try a chair in a quiet room by a window. Outside, you may prefer a park bench, a river bank, a lone hilltop, or an open field. Of course, a quiet house of worship works, too.

2. **Quiet your thoughts.** Easier said than done for most of us. Our thoughts are like a constant stream, a "tape" or "radio station" running all the time. It's futile to try to stop thinking. The more you resist thinking the more you'll *be* thinking. Instead, try some of these solutions:

- *Focus on your breathing,* using the strategy from the previous chapter.

- *Imagine your thoughts* are *a stream.* Picture them flowing by. Imagine yourself backing away from them and into a place of stillness and calm that exists apart from all noise and activity. As you allow your focus to drift toward the stillness, even inner-thought noise will recede.

- *Notice any sensations of relaxed calm* that flood your body, for instance, that wonderful "heaviness" in your shoulders, chest, or mid-section. Notice the "sense" of quiet you feel inside. *The more you can recognize and focus on these "target" sensations the better. They will become your "mark"—the state of being you want to return to—when anxiety tries to grip you again.*

- *When thoughts return, and they will, don't try to resist them.* Turn your attention back to the physical and/or interior sensations of calm. You may want to keep a pad and pen with you to capture important reminders such as appointments, phone calls, or tasks you need to remember...or quick insights. But resist the urge to journal.

3. **"Practice" quiet and calm.** Everyone experiences some anxiety. But for us, anxiety and related disorders are a threat to our health and well-being because they have become ingrained. They are our mind, body, or spirit's default mode.

For this reason, *it's imperative that we establish the experience of quiet calm at the deepest level of our being as possible.*

Set aside time as often as you can—I recommend 30 minutes daily, if possible—to practice inner quiet and calm. If 30 minutes *isn't* possible right now, start with a smaller block of time and expand it as you can. As you do this, you'll find yourself creating a sanctuary of inner solidity to return to wherever you are...a state of being that sensations and discomforts of anxiety cannot shake apart.

Strategy 4: Allow Your God to Have a "Makeover"

British author J.B. Philips wrote the classic book *Your God Is Too Small* many years ago. In it, he challenges us to reexamine and stretch our concepts about God, so that our views more closely match the wonder and mystery of the God who actually exists. Some of us who suffer spiritually based anxiety, also hold concepts of God, or how God views us and acts toward us, that need revising. In short, we've put "the wrong face" on God. We'll benefit when we discover that our God needs a serious makeover...and change our views about the character and nature of God.

Do This

1. **In the company of your spiritual confidant, or in a personal journal, explore your gut-honest answers to the following questions:**

- When I think of God, I think of... [*What's your description?*]

  _____

  _____.

- When I think about God's involvement in my everyday life, I think God

  _____ *is involved somehow.*

  _____ *is involved, but only in "big" or "important" matters.*

  _____ *is involved on some occasions...but which ones are a mystery to me.*

  _____ *is not involved at all...because God has bigger, better things to do, or God is not big enough to handle my problems.*

  _____ *has turned away from me because _____.*

- When I really need something, or when I'm in danger or in trouble, I believe God

  _____ *offers divine help, sometimes in "miraculous" or surprising ways.*

  _____ *wants me to struggle on my own, so I grow stronger and more capable.*

  _____ *doesn't see, or know, or care.*

  _____ *uses the hard things in life to show me just how little, unwise, wrong, or sinful I am...so I can see just how much I need to depend on God.*

- When I do something wrong (by my action or inaction) God is most likely to

  _____ *find a way to show me where I went wrong and help me understand how to correct my failings.*

  _____ *punish me...or let the worst happen to humiliate me.*

  _____ *keep anything bad from happening to me anyway, because God totally loves me.*

- When bad things happen in my life (and there is no human agency involved) it is

  _____ *God's fault.*

  _____ *the devil's fault.*

  _____ *probably my fault.*

  _____ *mostly a mystery.*

- When God looks at me, I believe God must feel

  _____ *warmth, kindness, love.*

  _____ *ashamed, like I am a failure.*

  _____ *disgust, loathing.*

_____ *angry.*

_____ *ready to abandon me.*

_____ *ready to throw me in hell.*

Certain beliefs about the fundamental character of God will pave the way for spiritually based anxiety. So will certain beliefs about God's level of involvement, the way we believe God will treat us when we need help or we've messed up, or our beliefs about God's view of us.

We experience anxiety when we believe God is fundamentally unhappy with us or ready to abandon, punish, or condemn us. Depending on how capable we feel of meeting life's challenges, we may also experience anxiety if we believe God lets us face struggles totally on our own. A fundamental uncertainty about God may also foster anxiety because we all need solid "spiritual ground" on which to stand when hard times come.

2. Begin the work of "balancing out" your beliefs about God, God's involvement in your life, and God's attitude toward you.

If you discover that your version of God is too legalistic and punishing...or too indifferent to struggle and pain...or too weak...or just too vague, you need to check in with other people who have spent time exploring "God questions." To do this you can:

- *Balance out your spiritual conversations.* Visit different Christian communities, and talk with other people about their experiences of faith.

- *Balance out your reading on spiritual subjects.* If you are from one faith tradition—say, Protestant and Reformed, read the writings of the early Church fathers and mothers, or the Catholic mystics. And vice versa. If your reading on the inner life consists only in books by post-modern philosophers or contemporary self-help books, for a change, read books by people who have a distinct faith and spiritual experience.

3. Learn to "approach" yourself with forgiveness. Many of us have internalized voices that judge us harshly. We can reproach ourselves unmercifully. We batter ourselves for breaking the rules and pushing the limits.

Letting our image of God go through a makeover means learning to approach ourselves and every one of our flaws and failures with a forgiving attitude. This is not about excusing—but it is about understanding and finding the way to change for the good. This attitude of forgiveness and love is the gift of Christian spirituality to the world.

Strategy 5: Embracing Change...and Reality

One of the most universal characteristics of the human spirit is that we all need stability. We begin life in a warm, tranquil, secure environment...and come out the chute grasping for a handhold and stable footing.

From that moment on, it's one long journey in search of ways to control this big reality we're passing through—one long attempt to wrap security and stability around us like pieces of spiritual clothing—while life keeps trying to rip it off and expose us.

We seek security and stability in many things, including *other people (or groups), possessions, money,* and *positions (at work or in the community).* We may seek security and stability purely in *ourselves* by becoming *strong* and *fit, capable, knowledgeable,* and *independent* so we can meet most of our own needs. Some of us build whole philosophies and lifestyles around the central purpose of isolating our weaknesses and vulnerabilities from the eyes of other people.

What we look to—what we depend on—as our source of inner security and stability is very important to our well-being. When that source of security and stability is threatened, or fails us, we experience trauma in the bedrock of our being. When our foundational views of reality are shaken, spiritually based anxiety is the result.

When we suffer anxiety, we can benefit by examining our foundational beliefs and understanding where our most fundamental

SPIRITUAL READING

〜

People who suffer from anxiety often find a great deal of spiritual relief in reading the scriptures. For centuries, Christian spiritual directors have recommended the practice of *lectio divina*, or "sacred reading" to solve various inner-life maladies...including anxiety.

In particular, many turn to the book of *Psalms* for spiritual buoyancy when anxiety sends its shock waves. I recommend that you read through these amazing writings, which reflect every possible inner state. Mark the passages that give your soul a sense of stability and peace, so you can turn to them when anxiety strikes. Here are a few to get you started:

Psalm 16	Psalm 23	Psalm 46
Psalm 18:1-6	Psalm 27:1-3	Psalm 57
Psalm 20	Psalm 31:1-5	Psalm 62:1-8

sense of well-being comes from. If we've made a habit of seeking stability from the wrong sources, we can readjust our inner life habits.

Do This

1. In the company of a spiritual confidant, or in a personal journal, explore your gut-honest responses to the following statements:

• My greatest source(s) of security and stability are:

___ my abilities, knowledge, talents, personality, or some other aspect of myself.

___ my body, and physical health and well-being.

_____ my husband/wife, boyfriend/girlfriend.

_____ my family, friends, coworkers, members of my spiritual community.

_____ my job or career.

_____ my performance (if I do well or do right, everything will work out fine).

_____ my home, possessions, or financial resources.

_____ my hopes and dreams for the future.

_____ my spiritual beliefs, or spiritual community.

_____ my relationship with God.

_____ I cannot identify a source of inner security, stability, or well-being.

• If I lost [*who* or *what*] I would be shaken to the core, and I don't know how I'd go on.

_____.

• If I lost [*who* or *what*], I would lose my faith.

_____.

2. Read through the statements, and your responses, again. This time, be aware of any "censors" that may have kept you from responding with absolute truthfulness. If necessary, switch off any inner screening devices and answer more honestly.

Many of us were trained as kids to say what other people want to hear. When it come to matters of faith we're still likely to give "the correct" doctrinal answer, or say what we think our spiritual friends or God wants us to say. *Getting out the truth can take work.*

3. Recognize sources of spiritual security and stability that are subject to change…and those that are not.

Our greatest disappointments, and our spiritually based anxieties, often come from the fact that we are looking for a reliable source of well-being that will never let us down. But as one wise spiritual teacher said, "Everything *beneath* heaven is subject to change...."

So here's the problem: We want a "fixed" and "sure" source of security and stability...but we rely on people and things that are subject to the same earthly forces of change that we are. As one spiritual writer said, "This is a good way to set yourself up to be let down by your false god." The result is anxiety.

Go through the list one more time, and place a check mark by the things you trust in for your greatest sense of security that are actually subject to the changing conditions of life on this planet.

4. Begin the process of transferring your trust to true sources of security and stability, ones that are not subject to change.

Some versions of spirituality act as if the spiritual life is an *arrival point*, not an *ongoing process* of deepening and maturing.

In one sense, the world we live in and the people we love are a great "laboratory" for learning how to deepen and mature in spirit. That's because they present us with the very condition our security- and control-driven selves do not want to face: *constant change.*

We mature in spirit by living out of a clearer understanding about the nature of life and reality. We deepen in spirit as we develop greater wisdom about how to live in relation to reality. And reality is all about *change.* We grow spiritually by learning to see the world as it really is, and at the same time by learning to live with grace and insight in the midst of changing and difficult realities.

Do This

1. Meditation #1: Seeing things the way they are.

Here are some observations about reality which, at first, may trigger sadness or anxiety. The more you meditate on them, the more they will become part of a more stable spiritual foundation. (You might call it the foundation of that spiritual sanctuary you're creating.) But once they become part of your working view of reality, they will actually begin to set you free from the anxiety that comes from looking for security and stability in a shifting world.

- *The things I rely on for my security are subject to change.*

- *The people I rely on are subject to change.*

- *I am subject to change, too.*

- *Even my understanding about God and ultimate realities is subject to change.*

Deep-level anxiety is the result when we try to hold on to a static view of things on one hand, hoping against hope that reality will be one way—when our experience tells us it is another way. Meditating on the changing nature of things gets us ready for the next step.

2. Meditation #2. Seeing that all change can have creative power.

For some of us, change represents a threat to our comfort and security and the destruction of the life we have arranged. We rarely glimpse the truth about our "religion" or "faith"—that it's not real faith at all, but a search for spiritual formulas that will make God do what we want God to do, which is work hard to protect the life we've arranged.

But as Joseph Campbell has observed, "We must be willing to let go of the life we have planned, so as to have the life that is waiting for us."

The problem is, as we've seen, change is inescapable—and most of us see change and its turmoil as only *destructive*. We say: "A bomb hit me." "It was like a tornado blew through." "I went through hell." If we want to manage deep anxiety we can learn to reenvision the forces of change, focusing on its other characteristic, which is *creativity*. We can meditate on and picture:

- *the "river" of time*…as its currents carry away certain people, places, things, and events.

- *the "seed" of our own spirit*…growing in all kinds of weather, passing through life's seasons, losing some things to the wind and wild, putting down deeper roots and new shoots, to become strong and steady…an evergreen…a tulip poplar… maybe an oak.

- *the natural rhythm of light and dark…warmth and cold…*the unstoppable, wondrous cycles of life and death, love and loss—those greater forces that can transform us into people of grace and wisdom.

- *the "hand of God" changing our lives…*sometimes taking away the old to make a place for the new.

- *the widening "space" inside…*that "sanctuary of quiet calm" within that life's changes and shakings cannot destroy.

Viewpoint is vital to life. People who have a narrow and tightly defined view of God, reality, and right and wrong are more susceptible to spiritual ailments such as anxiety. That's because God will not be shut in a box of anyone's theology. He reserves the right to keep surprising us all. People who learn to be flexible and allow for change and growth keep growing in faith and are more resilient when the beliefs, people, or things they rely on for security and stability are challenged.

Debra, who blamed God for "letting" her wonderful father die, says she benefited most from this strategy. "I realized that in my mind life was 'static.' Sure I was aware that *some* aspects of life change. But I didn't really have spiritual wisdom about the true nature of life on this planet. Everything changes. That's not necessarily *bad*, though it can be painful. It made a profound difference in me when I took a good look at reality and was able to say, 'Wonderful as this world is, and wonderful as my Dad was, only God is eternal.' I guess I'm a more 'philosophical' person than I knew. I *needed* that view of life to give me spiritual stability. Now I have a deeper peace about things than I ever had. It relieved the deep anxiety that was undermining my professional decision-making."

In Closing

My personal experience is that spiritual issues have a powerful energy, either for good or ill. We can live at odds with our true selves and never know it—until the anxiety generated in our core being sends shock waves into our mind and body, creating illness and making life miserable.

These issues, however, are among the toughest for us to face. Facing them may require us to have the courage to question beliefs and views on which we've based our whole lives and made our most important life choices.

As we close this chapter, I wish you the courage to reexamine the core issues of your life. I hope you will experience the resolution of your deepest conflicts, relieving the anxiety in spirit that makes you sick and keeps you from fully becoming who you were created to be.

5

The Food Factor

As we've noted, anxiety can originate from many sources. One such source, often overlooked, is food. It's true—what we eat can have a powerful effect on our moods, triggering anxiety. *Jerry* says, "When I eat certain foods it sends my anxiety through the roof." *Sheryl* is hypoglycemic, and when her blood-sugar level drops she becomes shaky, headachy, tired, and anxious.

Other people associate certain foods—or sometimes the very act of eating—with strong emotions. A friend who was mercilessly belittled for being fat in childhood has a terrible relationship with food today and can hardly put a bite of food in her mouth without triggering some level of anxiety.

Many of us, however, are not that aware of the effect foods or eating can have upon us. And so food and/or our relationship to eating work as "hidden" triggers.

We can benefit greatly by understanding "the food factor" in creating anxiety. This requires us to develop more self-awareness.

Strategy 1: Recognize Your Food–Mood Connections

When anxious energy is jolting through our body, we generally respond in one of two ways. Some of us *starve* and some of us *stuff.* Anxiety can drive us to down a half-gallon of ice cream…or a fifth of scotch. It can also cause our stomach to clench and refuse even a mouthful of food.

Likewise, eating over-salted, or high-fat food, or foods with certain additives, or foods that cause an allergic response, can send our anxiety level through the roof.

What are your *food–mood connections?* The better you understand the ways food and eating trigger anxiety, the better prepared you are to avoid food and situations that produce an anxious response.

Answering the sets of questions that follow will help you become more aware of your own food–mood connections. Given the fact that some of us feel ashamed or guilty about our eating habits, you may need to be aware that harsh, critical "voices" may make this exercise difficult. If this occurs, I encourage you to listen to *my* voice instead: *There is no one to blame—not even yourself—for what, when, why, or how you eat. Be at peace.*

- What *particular foods* do I reach for to calm or comfort or just distract myself when the emotions become strong?

  When I feel...

  —*restless* or *bored* I eat _____.

  —*irritated* or *angry* I eat _____.

  —*sad* or *depressed* I eat _____.

  —*anxious* I eat _____.

  —*numb* or *"flat"* I eat _____.

- What *situations* that involve eating (for example, the stress of holidays; parties where there are a lot of fat or sugary foods) tend to make me feel...

  —*restless* or *bored* _____

  —*irritated* or *angry* _____

  —*sad* or *depressed* _____

  —*anxious* _____

Strategy 2: Track Your Food–Moods

It's important to look at your whole *range of strong emotional responses to food and eating.* Why? Because strong emotions tend to change form inside us. Depending on our emotional wiring, we can start out feeling bored...or sad or depressed...and a while later find ourselves in the grip of anxiety...wondering, "How did I get here?" Most of us are subject to a kind of "emotional drift." We might eat a particular food, or eat in an uncomfortable setting...then go through a number of subtle (or not so subtle) emotional changes... and wind up engulfed in anxious energy.

Elena, for instance, happily looked forward to getting together with her extended family on weekends. She'd leave, however, feeling anxious and miserable. She'd also feel over-full and disgusted with herself. As she worked through the connections, she realized this: At almost every family gathering some loud argument erupted... she'd feel upset and eat to calm her jitters...and the food *would feel* comforting, but later the undealt-with anxieties returned *and* she felt sick to her stomach on top of it.

Ken ate whenever he felt irritated or angry. He felt angry a lot. The feel of food in his stomach was comforting. But soon the anger-turned-passive made another turn into anxiety. Because eating for comfort didn't solve the problem that made him angry in the first place, the real issues were still there, undealt with, and getting worse.

Eli loves oriental food. It took him awhile to establish the track of his anxiety attacks, but eventually he traced it back to the food additive *monosodium glutamate* (MSG), often used to flavor oriental dishes. What made it especially difficult was that the restaurant he frequented claimed they didn't add MSG to their food. But when Ken tried an elimination diet, and dropped oriental food from his menu for several weeks, the bouts with sudden anxiety ceased. (For more about "elimination diets" see page 92.)

If we want to change a habit, it helps to know its "track," from trigger-to-feeling, or feeling-to-action. Take time right now to think through and write down the track of any food–mood habits that create anxiety.

- *When I eat* (in this setting, at this time, with these people)

_____

_____

I can wind up feeling anxious.

- *When I am* (what physical state—tired? over-hungry?)

  _____

  _____

  I can wind up feeling anxious.

- *I feel* (name any of the various emotions you may also experience) _____

  _____

  and wind up feeling anxious.

Any time we learn more about the whole "life context" that creates our anxiety we make progress. Discovering the foods, the settings, and the emotional states that contribute to our anxiety can be an important step. When we understand our relationship to food and eating, we can prepare ourselves to handle anxiety-inducing situations.

Strategy 3: Find Healthy Alternatives for "Problem" Foods

Some foods create physical conditions that stress our body. When our body is stressed, emotional distress is a half-step away.

The truth is, just about any food can trigger a physical stress-response and send us down our own "track" to anxiety. This can happen when a particular food is hard to digest. So one person's easy-to-down bowl of oatmeal can be another person's digestive nightmare. We're all different. Also, keep in mind that overeating itself taxes the body and creates distress.

Some foods, however, are well-known for creating strong physical effects. Pay particular attention to your intake of the following foods that are known anxiety triggers. Just as important, make it part of your overall strategy to try the recommended alternatives.

Alcohol. Many people know that wines contain sulfites, which can cause severe headaches. But did you know that beer contains *tyramine*, a nitrogen compound that can irritate blood vessels in the brain? Beyond these problems, alcohol affects brain chemistry

∼

ANOREXIA, BULIMIA, AND BODY DYSMORPHIA

Researchers are divided over how to classify eating disorders such as *bulimia* and *anorexia*. Or how to classify the sometimes related disorder, *body dysmorphia*, whose sufferers have a distorted, unrealistic perception of their own body. Those who experience these disorders suffer terrible anxiety and emotional distress.

Seeking help for any of these disorders is not easy. Even *admitting* you have them is not easy. We're already struggling against voices inside that tell us there's "something wrong" or "bad" or "disgusting" about us. Admitting, "Yes, I have a problem" *seems* like giving up, giving in, and agreeing with that very negative voice that is already condemning us as "defective" or "worthless."

But it's *not* the same thing.

When you decide to seek help, you're not agreeing with the critical voices. What you're really saying is, "I don't know *why* I'm doing what I'm doing. But there is some reason for it. Maybe it's important to find out what that reason is and stop hurting myself. *Because no matter what I'm* doing, *I am a human being and a child of God. I'm worth helping and saving.*"

So while the self-care strategies in this book *will* help you, it's crucial for you to seek help from a healthcare professional who is experienced in treating these disorders. A garden variety counselor or psychologist, or a well-meaning friend or clergyman, will not do. You need professional, compassionate, *experienced* support.

When seeking help, ask these questions:

- What special training do you have in the treatment of this disorder?

- How many people have you treated who have this disorder? What kind of success rate have you seen?

- What kinds of other professionals do you work in association with in case I need a broader range of help? For example, psychiatrists, behavior therapists, clinics or support groups where this disorder is treated.

Bottom line: Don't be hesitant to interview the healthcare professional from whom you're seeking help. Don't be hesitant to switch care providers if their help isn't helping.

Your life, future, and well-being are on the line. Get help…and be sure it's the right help.

If you need assistance locating qualified professional help in your area, contact the Anxiety Disorder Association of America at (240) 485-1001 or online at: www.adaa.org.

∿

in general, also hormone production, blood pressure, digestion, and the lining of the urinary tract. And of course it affects mood.

"Moderation" is generally the key—but when it comes to alcohol and anxiety this is tricky. Too many people become physically or psychologically dependent on alcohol, saying, "I just need one drink…or two…to help me relax and calm down."

If you have been using alcohol to relieve anxiety it's very important that you stop doing this.

While we're on the matter of substances, the *nicotine* in tobacco is another substance we commonly use to help us relax and calm down. It's also horrendously addictive and can cause several life-threatening health conditions.

If you use tobacco…quit.

Alternatives: Natural juices and teas; nonalcoholic beer and wine; chewing gum; all the other strategies in this book.

Caffeine. Even a small amount of this powerful stimulant can send some of us over the edge. Not only does caffeine jolt our nervous and cardiovascular systems, the acid in coffee can create serious gastrointestinal problems. All told, caffeine triggers the anxiety response in more systems of the body than perhaps any other food substance.

Coffee, tea, colas—these drinks are obviously juiced-up with caffeine. But caffeine also hides in other foods such as chocolate and some non-cola soft drinks. There is even a small amount of caffeine in most "decaf" drinks. *Read labels.*

Alternatives: What if you love coffee and hate the flavor of decaf? First, try weaning yourself down to a cup…then a half-cup a day… sipped over a longer period of time. (When cutting back, or quitting, drink six to eight 8-ounce glasses of water a day to avoid "caffeine-withdrawal headaches.") If it's the comfort of a hot drink you're after, and you don't mind switching altogether, try green teas. They're rich in healthful nutrients, taste great, and have no caffeine.

Sugar. The average person in western culture consumes—in the lowest estimates—*20 teaspoons of sugar a day!* And if you drink non-diet soft drinks, the daily average is more than double that—about *50 teaspoons* of sugar! If you factor in corn sweeteners, and the sugar in most cereals, the amount of sugar eaten every day by the average person leaps again. Factor in cookies, ice cream, gum, and other "treats" and "comfort foods," and the amount soars until some of us are eating more than three or four full sugar-bowls of the white stuff every day.

White sugar causes blood-insulin levels to peak and drop rapidly. This can cause an emotional "high" and "low" that throws off our inner sense of balance and well-being. Then we need to eat something sugary to "offset" the anxious low we've dropped into…and welcome to mild addiction.

Alternatives: Stevia is a good and natural sugar substitute, which will not trigger the emotional rush and crash that white sugar delivers. Likewise, rice syrup, date sugar, and barley sugar are good alternatives. *Avoid* aspartame, saccharin, and products sweetened with them.

Salt. The sodium in salt plays a major role in affecting blood-pressure. Too much sodium also causes fluid retention, and we're better off keeping our bodies flushed.

Salt is another of those substances that is grossly overdone in the western diet. Like sugar, it has something of an addictive effect.

Yes, we need sodium in our diet, but there is plenty of sodium in many foods in their natural state. One 8-ounce glass of skim milk contains approximately 130 mgs. of sodium. Nonfat yogurt yields

150 mgs. per cupful. Just two ounces of tuna—or one sandwich-full—will deliver 250 mgs. of sodium.

Alternatives: Begin to use minimal salt on your foods...until you can cut out salting altogether. Buy low-salt products. Try salt-substitutes or experiment with dried herbs as flavoring. You will be amazed how much better your food tastes as you experiment with a diversity of flavors.

Strategy 4: Use an Elimination Diet

Other foods than those just listed can trigger anxiety. Sometimes additives in certain food products we eat may cause us problems, as well. Even if you suspect that a certain food may create physical stress leading to anxiety, detecting this for sure may be difficult.

The answer is to use an "elimination diet."

Do This

1. Make a list of all the foods you eat in a two-week period. This is fairly easy because most of us eat a relatively narrow variety—10 to 12 different foods.

Keep a second list of any unusual, or "occasional" foods you eat during this period, too.

Make a third list of additives in the prepared foods you eat, including preservatives, cooking oils, food colorings.

Create a fourth list of any and all supplements you take during this period.

2. Select one of the foods you eat most often and eliminate it from your diet for the two weeks. In particular, pay attention to any physical or mood changes. (Being cranky because you're not eating your favorite ice cream for two weeks doesn't count.)

3. Continue. At the end of two weeks, if you experience no changes you may want to add that food back into your diet. Then select another food, or a food additive, and eliminate it next.

Although this strategy is not difficult, it does take time, and it requires you to pay close attention to how you react after eating (or not eating) certain foods. Keep track of your reactions.

4. Create a Food–Mood Journal

Using a Food–Mood Journal is easy, and a great way to detect any reactions you might miss in an otherwise busy life. It's also a good way to create a record should you need to discuss your observations or questions with a healthcare professional.

Using a simple, spiral-bound notebook you can create your own journal, setting up the pages like this.

Food–Mood Journal

Week: 1/1 through 1/7

Eliminating: Caffeine (coffee and chocolate bars)

Physical Reactions:

1/1: Felt headachy today. Drank 6 glasses of water, and the headache went away.

1/2: No headache. Also, no chocolate "rush" followed by the usual "crash" that always makes me want to take a nap. I also noticed I was less jittery. But I got a little tired in the afternoon. (Maybe I should skip the 11:00 news and get to bed earlier?)

1/3: I was feeling really clear-headed and calm today. After lunch at an Italian restaurant, I noticed that all the salt in the spaghetti sauce made me unbelievably thirsty. I also felt a kind of pressure in my ears. Pretty sure my blood pressure jumped. (Better check this with the doctor.)

Emotional Reactions: This week I felt less "shaky" inside. *Much* more calm when stressful things occurred. Also, I didn't wake up after my "chocolate crash" naps feeling weird, out of sorts, and anxious. The salty spaghetti sauce thing was a surprise. Scary. I'm going to eliminate salt next, to see if that decreases my stress and anxiety level.

Eliminating, or greatly reducing your intake of problem foods is a precursor to the next strategy. This is not just about "taking things away." This is about creating a new eating plan that will help you experience a greater sense of physical and emotional well-being.

Strategy 5: Create a Balanced Diet

Any type of extreme diet can unbalance our body and, eventually, tip the scales on our emotional state. The thing is, most of us don't think of our diet as extreme. We'd probably say that we eat "a typical western diet."

The truth is, the typical western diet can be called extreme because it's highly unbalanced. Besides being loaded with the stress-producing substances we've discussed, the average western diet is high in all the very things that stress the body and contribute to mood swings. This includes: cholesterol-producing proteins, saturated fats, and a massive over-abundance of simple carbohydrates, all of which send our hormonal systems reeling.

Most of us eat such an unbalanced diet habitually that we have no idea how much it's detracting from our overall health and eroding our emotional state.

Alternative: Many doctors and nutritionists today recommend that we eat a diet in which each meal is comprised of :

- 40 percent complex carbohydrates—from fruits, vegetables, or legumes.

- 30 percent lean protein—from fish, poultry, free-range chicken eggs, or plant sources such as soy, barley, brown rice, oats, quinoa.

- 30 percent fat—*beneficial* fats such as the fat from flax, hemp, olive, and sesame oils, and also the essential fatty acids found in fish oils.

The best and most widely used 40-30-30 balanced-eating plan is "the Zone Diet," researched and formulated by Dr. Barry Sears. To get started, read *Mastering the Zone* or, if you prefer a vegetarian diet, try *The Soy Zone,* both written by Dr. Sears.

The great thing about "the 40-30-30 diet" is that it keeps our insulin and other hormonal levels balanced. Therefore, it keeps our energy levels on an even keel, and that helps keep us emotionally in-balance, as well. As a result, we're less susceptible to powerful mood swings, including the ones that can toss us right into all-out anxiety.

"HIDDEN" FOOD ADDITIVES

〜

When it comes to prepared foods, here's one imperative we can't afford to ignore: *Read the labels.*

Some of us scan labels for calorie or fat content but overlook the ingredients and additives that help create serious health problems. Even words like "Lite" or "Low Sodium" on the front of the label may mean very little when we turn the package over and read the contents list. We all need to be more aware of food contents that contribute to physiological stress and trigger emotional distress.

Look for:

- **Sodium.** Even a can of so-called "healthy" soup contains nearly *40 percent* of the recommended daily allotment of sodium.

- **"Sweeteners."** In most foods, this means "corn sweeteners," which cause those unwanted peaks and drops in our insulin levels.

- **"Natural Flavorings."** Unfortunately, this is the way some manufacturers get around listing what's really in their product. "Natural flavorings" often means monosodium glutamate (MSG). If MSG causes problems for you be cautious when you see this on a label.

- **BHA, Nitrites, and Sulfites.** These substances, commonly used to retard spoilage, can trigger headaches, migraines, and mood-fluctuations.

A Final Word of Encouragement

Altering our diet is one of the most difficult changes we can make. But the truth is, it's one of the most beneficial things we can do for our health and well-being.

Most people fail when it comes to changing what they eat for one simple reason: They try to make too great a change too quickly. Trying to switch to a whole new way of eating, or even to totally eliminate a food that causes us problems, is a plan that has a lot going *against* it. That is to say, most of us grossly underestimate *force of habit.*

Rather than try to change a lifelong, habitual way of eating in a day, or a week, or even a month, you'll be more successful if you build a transitional eating plan.

1. Eat one meal a day that follows the 40-30-30 diet plan described in this chapter. Make sure it includes foods from all three of the beneficial food groups mentioned.

2. In one month, add a second balanced meal. In this month, also begin to eliminate any foods that contribute to your anxious state.

3. *Two months* later, switch the third meal. If you feel ready to do this sooner, of course, go for it.

4. In one more month, make changes in your snacking habits. Minimize high-fat, sugary, white-flour-based treats. Keep delicious fresh and dried fruits handy, also low- and nonfat yogurt and ice cream.

In just four months you can remake your whole eating plan. If you do this, I can guarantee you'll experience tremendous benefits in your personal energy level, and in your emotional sense of stability and well-being.

6

Working Out Anxiety

A nxiety is a state of being we usually associate with our thoughts and emotions. Our first response, generally speaking, is to find ways to resolve anxious thinking or spiritual conflicts. Seldom do we consider that anxiety and its related disorders can have a physiological foundation, as well.

We can see this easily when we look at the effects of anxiety: Breathing gets shallow, our heart beats wildly, muscles clench. As we've seen, anxiety can also be generated by our physical reactions, for instance, when certain foods or eating patterns trigger hormonal or gastrointestinal reactions.

But there is more to this matter. Anxiety is such a strong sensation it can become ingrained in our physiology. We can develop such a strong anxiety-response that almost any challenge or strong emotional shift triggers our body to respond with the symptoms of anxiety.

Tom discovered, for instance, that life could present him with even the most positive circumstances—a big promotion and raise, a Caribbean vacation—and still his anxiety would cause his body to shake until he was soaked with perspiration. And sometimes the smallest challenge, like getting to the post office by 5:00 P.M. to mail a letter, made his hands moist with nervous anxiety.

In short, anxiety can be programmed into our nervous system and muscle fibres.

The good news is that we can reverse our body's anxiety-response by creating new and relaxing physical habits and find our way to a calmer, freer, living space. The truth is, when every impulse is shouting, "Stop breathing! Freeze!" *getting physically active* is one of the best things we can do to loosen anxiety's grip.

For this reason, creating a healthy, physical action plan plays a crucial part in anxiety relief.

Knowing When to Challenge...and When to Distract

In Chapter 2, we looked at an important overall strategy, which is knowing how to *challenge* life-dominating anxiety. Meeting the source of your anxious feelings and countering them from a place of inner calm and stability is a huge step in overcoming this uncomfortable condition.

The other aspect of anxiety relief, however, is knowing when to *distract* yourself from anxiety.

To this point, some of the strategies discussed in other chapters—for instance, breath work and shifting our focus—are useful in distracting us when we're over our heads with anxiety.

The importance of having *strategies that distract us* is twofold:

- *they help us "step away" from anxious inner-space quickly.*

- *they give us a strong experience of calm that empowers us mentally to go back to and face the anxiety trigger in a more stable state.*

In this chapter, we want to look at more of the body-boosting strategies we can use to literally step away from anxiety. These strategies also—

- *flush our muscle tissues of acids, relieving stored physical tension.*

- *balance our hormonal output by releasing hormones that heal and relax us, countering the effects of the stress-hormones released by anxiety.*

Without a good workout plan you can become, literally, an anxiety battery. That is, you carry around in your physical being the stored tension that contributes to the discomfort and distress of anxiety.

"Working Out" Your Anxiety

The strategies in this section are arranged from *low-*, to *moderate-*, to *greater-intensity* workouts. The truth, of course, is that any form of physical activity that holds our attention can provide an anxiety-relieving workout. Those described here, however, require no special skill or equipment.

The *low-intensity strategies* can be done even if your fitness level is low. Those of *moderate* intensity are especially useful if you need greater distraction or have just a bit of free time. The *greater-intensity strategies* are for those of us who need and/or enjoy a more demanding physical outlet.

You should try as many of these strategies as possible. Even if you're a more active person, you may not have time or be in a place to engage in one of the more physically demanding strategies. (Stretching is a great way, for instance, to ease anxiety when you're stuck on a plane or in an office.) Likewise, you may start out needing to use just the easier strategies and then find it helpful to increase your activity level…or you may just get more fit and come to love the focus and peace that comes after an intense workout!

Whatever your current situation, it's important to have a range of distraction strategies built into your overall plan for anxiety management.

Strategy 1: Make Your Workout a Priority

Working out is one of those things we *mean* to do…and we know it's important. *But…*

But everything else takes priority. While our body is crying out for health, anxiety-relief, and fitness, most of us give our energies to everything and everyone else. Then we crash in front of the TV or handle household duties till we drop. If we're going to take seriously our need to manage physiologically based anxiety we need to be proactive.

Do This

- **Create a monthly plan.** Buy an inexpensive planner. For many of us, exercise is such a luxury—or torture—that if we

OBSESSIVE EXERCISING

～

For some of us who suffer anxiety—especially those of us with eating disorders and body dysmorphia—obsessive exercising is sometimes a problem. We may exercise because we're anxious about our physical appearance or because we feel lonely or isolated or sad or angry...or just to "out distance" anxiety itself.

While we seldom think of those who aggressively pursue physical fitness as candidates for anxiety attacks, the man or woman who lives in the gym and is "ripped" may actually be suffering from anxieties that are driving him or her to exercise obsessively.

Obsessive exercising abuses our bodies, erodes our relationships, and can actually endanger our health. Obsessive exercising is distraction *in excess*. We literally do not stop running, and so we avoid facing the source of our anxiety...let alone learn how to challenge it.

If you are exercising obsessively, or in excess, you should seek the help of a healthcare professional.

don't plan for it, it won't happen. Workout time needs to be nonnegotiable.

- **Set aside some time each day for a light to moderate workout.** Choose three alternative time-slots—morning, midday, and evening. That way, if one time-slot is taken by an interruption, you have alternatives. We need this because, when some urgency robs our exercise time it's too easy to think, "Today's time is blown. Guess I can't exercise until tomorrow."

- **Set aside a minimum of 1 hour once a week for a more intense workout. If possible, work up to three 1-hour sessions a week.** If you have not exercised in some time, you will want to build up to this over a period of several months.

Consulting a healthcare professional before starting a more strenuous workout routine will give you the heart and blood-pressure information you need to exercise at the intensity for your age and physical condition.

• **Set aside time at least once a month for a longer period of physical activity you consider fun and relaxing.** Not all exercise should be about grunting and sweating. Find both outdoor and indoor activities that are very physical, so you can enjoy yourself and give your body a boost throughout the year.

Bottom line: *Wanting* to work out isn't enough. *Making a commitment* isn't enough. *Taking charge of your schedule, planning exercise into your life,* and *doing* it is the right beginning.

Strategy 2 (Low Intensity): Stretching and Massage

Wait a minute—this section is about working out, right?

That's right. And both stretching and massage are excellent ways to work out the stress that stores itself in our muscles. Both are excellent light forms of exercise, especially for beginners and those of us starting over.

Stretching

The great thing about stretching is that you don't need to buy anything. Stretching is probably one of the most under used anxiety-relief techniques, and it offers great benefits. For a basic stretching workout that releases tension from those "anxiety batteries" you know as muscles.

Do This

1. **Extend your arms out in front of you. Clasp your hands as if gripping a handle.** Using your right arm, slowly draw your left arm up and to the right—to the "2 o'clock" position. Pull with enough effort to feel the muscles around your left shoulder blade and upper

back as they stretch. Hold for 20 to 30 seconds, breathing deeply. Relax and repeat.

Do the same for the benefit of your right side.

This stretch "opens up" your back.

2. Extend your arms out in front of you again. Hold your hands together "prayer-style." Slowly raise both hands together toward the sky. When you reach the "12 o'clock" position, let your arms spread open wide enough to feel your chest and abdominal muscles stretch…as your arms come down to your sides. Relax and repeat.

This stretch opens up your upper midsection, allowing for deep-cleansing breathing.

3. Create a circle in front of you with your arms and clasped hands. Maintaining the circle, rotate your arms to the right, until your clasped hands are behind your hips. Feel the muscles in your abdomen, left hip, and lower back stretch. Hold for 20 seconds.

Relax and repeat.

Do it again, circling back to the left.

Stretching these muscles opens up your lower-midsection, allowing for even deeper breathing and releasing tension in the lower back.

4. (Standing.) Keep your knees firm, but not stiff. Let your arms hang loose. Slowly bend toward the floor. Don't worry about touching the floor, just *relax into this stretch.* Hold for 20 seconds…come back up *slowly.* Relax and repeat.

This stretches the gluts, the hamstrings, and the tendons all along the back of your legs.

5. (Standing.) Rest your left hand against a wall. Raise your left foot behind you and clasp it with your right hand. Gently pull your left leg back, feeling the quadricep muscles stretch. Hold for 20 seconds. Relax and repeat.

Do it again for the benefit of the right leg.

The large muscles of the legs are sometimes referred to as "the second heart" because they help pump blood through the lower body. You really want to keep these muscles strong and flexible!

*A **note about necks.** Never* roll your head in a circle to loosen neck muscles. This can damage the delicate disks between your cervical vertebrae. Instead, *gently tilt* your head from *side to side,* and *front to back.*

Massage

We're just discovering the health benefits of *massage,* a strategy other cultures have used in healing regimens for centuries. Deep-muscle massage is a great alternative way to stimulate the release of tension-causing hormones and acids from the muscles.

Do This

1. **Contact a local LMT (Licensed Massage Therapist).** Most people find it uncomfortable to be touched by a stranger. Give yourself time to relax into the therapy and enjoy it.

HEALING TOUCH

∼

There is a physiological reason why *touch* has the power to help heal us.

When we touch, the skin-to-skin sensation is so powerful it triggers the production of oxytocin, a hormone released by the pituitary gland. This hormone offers the body amazing benefits, physically and psychically.

Physically, oxytocin causes muscles to relax. It's such a powerful relaxant that its release during childbirth, for instance, can cause the uterine muscles to relax faster, speeding up delivery. (So the next time you're in labor, or your wife is, use massage to help speed things along naturally!) The release of oxytocin also creates a powerful, all-over, feeling of serenity.

Massage is an important strategy to use when you are down…or anxious!

2. Or obtain an illustrated massage guide, and work with a partner. I recommend, *Massage for Dummies: A Reference for the Rest of Us* (1999), by Steve Capellini and Michel Van Welden.

Strategy 3 (Low to Moderate Intensity): Walking as Therapy

Walking is a great way to get physical exercise *and* work anxiety out of your body. It's actually great therapy.

You'll want to walk where you can move along freely, at a low to moderate pace.

Do This

1. **Choose two or three walking routes.** Pick a shorter route (10 minutes), one that's mid-range (20 minutes), and a longer course (30+ minutes). This will give you options, depending on the time you have available.

2. **Set out, leaving your anxieties behind.** It will help to use the mental anxiety relief strategies *before* you set out. It may help, for instance, to have a mental "ritual," like the following:

Tell yourself, "My anxiety will start to [shrink, dissolve, dissipate, be taken into God's hands] when I [walk out the door, leave the property]."

3. **Refocus on your breathing…or on the world around you.** Shifting your focus to something, somewhere, outside yourself is another aspect of this strategy. The more you're able to focus on the solid, stable outer world, the more you distract yourself from the shaky, "coming apart" sensations of anxiety.

4. **Pick up the pace and increase your heart-rate.** Reach a good rhythm in your stride, one that's aggressive enough to elevate your heart-rate and deepen your breathing. *This stimulates the parasympathetic nervous system, which releases those relaxation and healing hormones.*

5. Allow yourself to cool down slowly. As your walk comes to an end, slow your pace so that you experience a good 5- to 10-minute cool-down. After elevating your heart-rate, it is not a good idea to sit or lie down immediately. Let your pulse and respiration come back to normal first.

HITTING THE TARGET

∾

You don't need to invest in an electronic monitor to know your heart-rate. You can easily check your pulse by placing the index and middle fingers of your right hand on your left medial artery – which is that "blue pencil line" at the base of your left thumb at the cuff-line.

Below are target "working heart-rates" you can shoot for if you want to achieve a good aerobic workout. "Hitting" your target heart-rate for at least 30 minutes, three times a week, is an excellent health objective. At the lower end, you'll be burning fat. At the upper end, you'll be giving your heart a great workout. *Caution:* If you're out of shape, ask your healthcare professional what heart-rate range is best for you.

Age Range

25 117 to 156 beats per minute (20 to 26 beats per 10 seconds)

35 111 to 148 beats per minute (19 to 25 beats per 10 seconds)

45 105 to 140 beats per minute (18 to 23 beats per 10 seconds)

55 99 to 132 beats per minute (17 to 22 beats per 10 seconds)

65+ 93 to 124 beats per minute (16 to 21 beats per 10 seconds)

Strategy 4 (Moderate Intensity): Nonimpact Aerobics and Yoga

Nonimpact Aerobics

Nonimpact Aerobics (NIA) is a great workout experience that combines stretching with fluid motions. This exercise was created to be easy on the joints, while still elevating the heart-rate. The routines are described as a blend of several activities including aerobics, ballet, muscle toning, and weight training.

NIA is a fantastic way to ease the tension of anxiety. It increases metabolism and releases the hormones and neurotransmitter chemicals in the brain that cause us to experience calm. NIA also encourages you to develop a positive frame of mind, which adds to its list of anxiety-relieving benefits.

Do This

1. Check local community centers, gyms, or health clubs to sign up for NIA classes.

2. As you work through the NIA routines, focus on positive thoughts and spiritual truths that lift your mind and ease spiritual tension.

Yoga

Yoga is an 8,000-year-old practice that's now taking the world by storm. There are several types of yoga, and most health clubs and gyms offer courses.

Many yoga courses are taught with a modern twist. That is, *they're offered purely for the exercise benefit,* though some instructors still bring in the Eastern philosophies associated with yoga. Obviously, when dealing with anxiety, you should avoid types of yoga that increase your sense of personal tension. For instance, you may wish to avoid classes that emphasize philosophies you don't agree with. You may also wish to avoid "Hot Yoga," which is yoga practiced in a very hot room.

Overall, though, the health benefits and calming effects of yoga exercise have contributed to its being kept alive for eight millennia.

Do This

1. **Check out yoga classes in your area.** Ask about the focus of the class, and about the level. Some types of yoga are suited for beginners, and some are more strenuous and require a higher degree of fitness.

Strategy 5 (Intense): Aerobics and Weight Training

If you're in that phase of life when the fact that you were once in shape is a pleasant memory, it's important to have a physical checkup before beginning any kind of intense exercise.

Aerobics

Those of us who have been less active should ease into aerobic workouts. If you're reasonably fit, though, aerobic exercise offers a great channel for energy that would otherwise be channeled into anxiety. Aerobics classes are easy to find and there is a variety to choose from—from standard routines, to step aerobics, to "dance-r-cise."

Do This

1. **Visit several types of aerobics classes to decide which type you prefer.**

2. **Be sure the instructor is attuned to your needs, which include:**

- beginning with a slower, warm-up pace
- moving through a variety of paces and exercises
- ending with a slower, cool-down pace

Weight Training

No longer is weight training the realm of the young "hard bodies." Men and women of all ages are discovering the physical and mental-health benefits. Because it requires careful attention and focus, it's an excellent "distraction" *and* it releases pent-up energy, while toning and slimming your body. (What's not to like?)

Good weight training requires know-how. Otherwise, it's easy to injure yourself and to waste a lot of energy with little benefit.

Do This

1. Check out health clubs and gyms in your area. Many facilities will have a free-weights section *and* weight machines. Be sure the facility you choose has both.

2. Use weight machines first…and graduate to free weights. The benefit of weight machines is that they help you build muscles that support your joints. Too often people jump over to the free-weights side of the gym without building good joint-strength and stability first, and that's when injuries occur. Give yourself time on the machines. When you switch to free weights, take more time to build from lighter to heavier lifting.

3. Get help from a trainer. Many health clubs have "attendants"—people who hang around wearing tee-shirts with the club's monogram. They can tell you what each machine is used for. *These people are not necessarily trainers.*

Bona fide trainers have had professional instruction and are credentialed. They can tell you *how* to use the weight machines and free weights in the proper way, and they can help you create a physical workout that's right for you, given your age, current level of fitness, and health goals. Most trainers hire out by the hour, so you can set up just one session to get yourself going or set up, say, a monthly meeting to review your progress and alter your workout routine as needed.

4. Chart your progress, and reward yourself for gains. Maybe you're not trying to become a world-class bodybuilder, but keeping track of your gains is a great way to boost your self-esteem and reinforce the positive-focused, healthy habit you're creating. Remember to reward yourself—say, with new workout clothes—as an added incentive.

In Closing

Just about everything in our culture seems bent *against* us getting the healthy physical workout we all need.

But if you're dealing with anxiety, getting into a regular physical discipline is one of the very best things you can do to direct pent-up physical energy and inner tension in a healthy direction. Not only will exercise give you the mental distraction you need to help you "step away" from anxiety and the physiological boost of an elevated metabolism, you'll experience the serene afterglow that comes from expending energy. You'll sleep better, too.

7

Natural Supplements

Some of the supplements discussed in this chapter are known to cause negative reactions in the body when taken in combination with prescription medications. Some are also known to cause negative reactions when taken in combination with other supplements.

Be advised: *Scientific testing of natural supplements is still ongoing. Therefore, it is not possible at this time to list all the possible contraindications that may occur after taking natural supplements.*

When using natural supplements to treat anxiety, panic attacks, or anxiety disorders you should do so in consultation with a healthcare professional.

Always notify your physician and pharmacist if you are using supplements in combination with prescription drugs.

S ome healthcare professionals discount the use of natural supplements in their treatment of anxiety, panic attacks, and anxiety disorders. Many doctors, for instance, note that natural supplements are not regulated or tested by government agencies, and therefore purity is in question. They also cite the fact that in laboratory tests, random samplings of some supplements have shown that the substance named on the label doesn't even show up in some of the capsules inside the bottle. How can you guard against side effects, doctors argue, or ensure that you're actually taking the supplement you're paying for?

Sadly, the same can be asked when it comes to prescription medications. According to a 1998 article in the *Journal of the American*

Medical Association (JAMA), 106,000 deaths and *2 million* severe reactions to prescription drugs occur every year in the United States alone, making side effects the *fourth leading cause of death* in America.* And of course there are many more side effects that go unreported, though they create long-term damage in the prescription-drug user. As one set of researchers put it: "Any drug, no matter how trivial its therapeutic actions, has the potential to do harm."†

When taking medications for anxiety it's important to ask, "What are the side effects I might experience from taking this drug?" Doctors often avoid discussing side effects out of a concern that they may plant suggestions in the mind of a patient (especially an already anxious one) and, therefore, create more anxiety or even trigger a psychosomatic occurrence of those side effects. But because our health is at stake, we need to have as much information as possible when we're taking potent substances into our bodies.

When treating some forms of anxiety, especially panic attacks and anxiety disorders, avoiding pharmaceuticals may not be an option. If you need intervention, don't be afraid of drug-therapy. Instead, ask questions and be armed with good information. Anxiety-intervention medication may be what you need to get you through the worst times.

But once you've gotten through those times when anxiety is crippling, you may want to seek therapeutic support from natural supplements. They are very effective, and may be a better choice if you need anxiety relief over a longer period of time. Some anxiety sufferers taper down their medications while building up to a therapeutic dose of natural supplements. If you keep open communication with your healthcare professional and pharmacist, you can avoid any harmful drug-supplement reactions. In this way, it may be possible in some cases to bring the therapeutic level of a natural supplement to a point that you're able to back down, or back off, prescription drugs altogether.

---

* J.P. Lazarou, BH, P.N. Corey, "Incidence of adverse drug reactions in hospitalized patients: a meta-analysis of prospective studies," *Journal of the American Medical Association,* 1998; 279(15):1200-5.

† A.G. Gilman, T.W. Rall, A.S. Nies, P. Taylor, *The Pharmacological Basis of Therapeutics* (Pergammon Press, 1996).

While drugs help with quick intervention, in the long-term, using natural supplements offers a more promising alternative… along with some very important health benefits.

Anxiety-Relief Benefits

Natural supplements are very effective in treating anxiety and its related disorders. Because they act in a gentler manner, slowly building up to a therapeutic dose, they can be used safely over a long period of time.

Several factors make natural supplements appealing when it comes to anxiety relief. Mainly:

- *Natural supplements do not cause the unwelcome side effects that come with some of the strong anti-anxiety medications, such as flattened emotions, weight gain, over-drowsiness, and the repression of sexual energy.*

- *While they are effective as mood-enhancers, bringing a sense of calm and balance, most natural remedies don't put us in danger of becoming drug-dependent.*

Along with these pluses, natural supplements offer great health benefits to our whole body—as you'll discover in the descriptions mentioned in this chapter. Supplements can play an important part in managing your anxiety, panic attacks, and anxiety disorders.

Let's take a walk through a "virtual health food store," where you can browse over some of the most popular, natural supplements that are recommended to relieve life-dominating anxiety.

A Small Apothecary
of Anxiety Relief Remedies
～～～

From the Amino Acid Shelf

Certain amino acids are necessary to help the brain function well. When the level of these amino acids is too low, our brains can "work against us" by absorbing *neurotransmitters*—those are the chemicals that assist the nerves of the brain as they send signals from one part of the brain to another. It's believed at this time that anxiety disorders can result when the brain has reabsorbed too much of the neurotransmitter *serotonin*.

Taking certain amino acids can slow the brain's absorption of its neurotransmitter chemicals, including serotonin. This leaves more serotonin available for normal brain functioning, leading to a decrease in anxiety. Amino acids can be helpful in the treatment of anxiety and anxiety disorders.

• *GABA* (Gamma Amino Butyric Acid) is an amino acid derivative that acts as a neurotransmitter chemical in the brain. It helps keep the brain's metabolism in balance. It can have a calming effect, like Valium or Lithium, but without the serious side effects…such as potential addiction.

Caution: The recommended dose is 200 milligrams, four times a day. However, too much GABA can actually cause anxiety. Careful monitoring of your intake of GABA, with professional guidance, is recommended. Notify your healthcare professional if you want to take GABA and you are taking Histadine and/or amino acid L-Tryptophan, because overuse of these substances in combination will have adverse effects.

Important Note: GABA is sometimes taken in combination with Vitamin B-6 (200 milligrams three times a day) and Chromium Picolinate (200 milligrams, once a day). In this combination, B-6 and Chromium Picolinate enhance GABA's absorption and effectiveness.

From the Herb Shelf

The use of herbal remedies is becoming widespread. Some would say *too* common. While they have a reputation for being "gentler" because they're "more natural," herbs are potent and can be misused.

You should use care when preparing to take herbs because herbs *are* strong medicines. *Read labels. Buy only from quality manufacturers. Know all the herbs included in a given product. Be aware of the effect they can have on you. If you do not recognize an herb, and know its effect, avoid it.* As always, *notify your healthcare professional and pharmacist if you're using herbs, as some can react negatively when taken in combination with prescription drugs.*

Once you become knowledgeable, herbal remedies can become an important part of your overall anxiety-relief plan. Here are some of the herbs you will find effective.

- *Barberry* (also known as *Oregon Grape*). This potent herb is often used to treat the stomach upset created by anxiety. It's also effective as a mild sedative. Barberry is available in capsules.

  Caution: Pregnant women should not take Barberry, as it can stimulate uterine contractions. Because of its sedative effects, you should not use Barberry in conjunction with Ativan, Valium, or Xanax.

- *Catnip.* You will experience a mildly relaxing effect from this pleasant member of the mint family. It also relieves nausea. Catnip is taken in tea or extract forms.

- *Chamomile.* Anxiety can produce terrible physical side effects, from stomachaches to colitis. And of course it can rob us of sleep. No single ingredient has been identified to account for the therapeutic benefits of this wonderful herb, and yet it is famed for easing gastrointestinal problems and promoting sound sleep. Chamomile comes loose, for making tea, and also in capsules and extract form.

  Note: Sometimes people with weed allergies—ragweed in particular—experience reactions to Chamomile.

- *Cramp Bark.* This herb has a more pleasant name: *Black Haw. Lydia Pinkham's Vegetable Compound,* one of the most popular women's medicines of the nineteenth and early twentieth centuries, was based on this herb. Its legendary effects as a muscle relaxant came to us through Native American tradition. Its overall anti-stress effects are wonderful. Call it Black Haw if that will help you feel better about using it. Cramp Bark/Black Haw is taken as an extract.

- *Kava.* Used for centuries in Polynesian cultures, this herb has gained a generally good reputation throughout the Western health-care community because its anxiety-reducing properties can be as effective as benzodiazepine drugs like Ativan, Valium, and Xanax. It's a powerful mood elevator. Kava can be taken in several forms—as a tea, in juice, in capsules, and in extract.

  Caution: This herb has caused some concern recently, though it appears that the problems associated with it were caused by overuse or because it was used without caution in combination with pharmaceuticals. (In one known case, Kava seems to have heightened the effect of a benzodiazepene drug, inducing a non-fatal coma.) Kava should not be taken by individuals with Parkinson's Disease. It should not be taken if you use alcohol or prescription sedatives.

- *Lemon Balm.* Folklore reveals that this herb has been used for centuries to relieve agitation and to induce sleep. Its greatest effects are felt in about a week. Lemon Balm is taken in tea, capsule, and extract forms.

- *Passionflower.* When this flower was first found, the three stiles inside its bright-red petals reminded its discoverers of the three nails that held Christ to the cross—hence, the name. It is widely used in Europe in the treatment of anxiety, nervous exhaustion, and insomnia. Passionflower can be taken as a tea, in capsules, and in extract form.

  Caution: This herb is not recommended for pregnant women unless its use is approved by a healthcare professional. Because it can cause drowsiness, avoid driving and operating heavy equipment. Allergic reactions and asthma have been reported in rare instances.

- **Rhodiola.** Many of us know about Siberian Ginseng (*eleu. senticosus*) and its whole-body tonic effects. But Rhodiola is qui. becoming a widely used and important adaptogen, too. Adaptogens are known as "super tonics" because they act upon every system of the body to increase resistance to physical, emotional, and chemical stressors. Rhodiola increases the production of serotonin in the brain, helping to bring a deep calm.

  Like Siberian Ginseng, Rhodiola is best used on a long-term basis, to raise your base-line stress-resistance level. Rhodiola is available in capsules and tablets. You can use the dried-leaf form if you prefer to make a fragrant, comforting, and healing tea.

- **St. John's Wort.** Widely used to treat anxiety and depression, researchers believe the active compounds in this herb—hypericin, pseudohypericin, and hyperforin—may assist the neurotransmissions in the brain. This may be the reason for its definite antianxiety effects. It can take up to two weeks to experience the benefit of St. John's Wort. St. John's Wort can be taken as a tea, in capsules, and in extract form.

  Note: *You should not take St. John's Wort if you are using MAO inhibitors. This herb does not react well with certain protease inhibitors. It's also known to cause skin hypersensitivity during sun exposure, so extra protection is advised. St. John's Wort may affect the metabolism of Coumadin, Clozaril, Elavil, Haldol, Theo-Dur, Tofranil, Zyflo, and Zyprexa.*

- **Valerian.** European doctors have long used Valerian to cure nervous disorders and panic attacks. Its effects are felt in 30 minutes to an hour. If you take a large dose late in the day, it can help you experience sound sleep, but you are likely to wake up groggy the next day. To avoid this, and for long-term use, build up to the dose that works for you, without causing the "hang over." Valerian can be taken in capsule and extract forms.

  Caution: *Valerian interacts with barbiturate drugs. If you are using benzodiazepine drugs like Ativan, Valium, and Xanax, you should*

BUYING HIGH-QUALITY SUPPLEMENTS

~

How do you know you're getting quality, when you're buying herbs, vitamins, and/or minerals?

Here are two ways you can check out the supplement manufacturers you're buying from.

- *Dietary Supplement Quality Initiative:* DSQI reviews natural supplements and makes its findings available to the general public. Read up on the latest supplement news on their website: **www.supplementquality.com**. If you can't find a review of the supplement(s) you're interested in, you may wish to call them at (617) 734-4123.

- *ConsumerLab.com.* This website posts the findings of dozens of independent labs that purchase supplements off-the-shelf, just like you do, and then test them. They test for purity, the accuracy of the information on the label, and consistency of dosage capsule-for-capsule. Candid results are free to you.

not use Valerian. Use of this herb is not recommended during pregnancy. It can also affect the metabolism of Coumadin, Clozaril, Elavil, Haldol, Theo-Dur, Tofranil, Zyflo, and Zyprexa.

From the Hormone Shelf

- *Melatonin.* If anxiety is disturbing your sleep, you need to know about melatonin, an effective and natural sleep-aid. This hormone is manufactured in the brain, using the neurotransmitter chemical serotonin, a substance responsible for, among other things, determining mood. Melatonin plays an important role in regulating the body's internal clock, and so it helps to control periods

of sleep and wakefulness. Normally, melatonin is releas___
pineal gland, at the base of the brain, as evening darkness falls,.
is suppressed by the return of morning light. During stressful, anxious periods, however, its production is greatly disrupted—and
this is what affects our ability to fall asleep and experience deep,
REM sleep, which is essential to our well-being. Melatonin can be
taken in doses of 3 mgs., 20 minutes before your desired bedtime.

*Caution: Though melatonin is widely used and generally considered
safe, you should consult with your physician before using it, especially
if you are pregnant or suffering an auto-immune condition or depres-
sive disorder.*

From the Mineral Shelf

• *Calcium, Magnesium, and Potassium.* Because stress is such a part
of most of our lives, the calcium, magnesium, and potassium in
our foods is often not enough to support the body's need for these
important minerals. In therapeutic doses, all three work to release
tension from the muscles and have a calming effect on emotions.
Potassium, additionally, supports the adrenal glands, which produce anti-stress hormones. These three minerals should be taken
together, and they're often sold in combination. Calcium can be
taken in 1000 mg. doses daily. It should be taken in its chelate form,
so it can better combine with magnesium and potassium. Magnesium can be taken in 1000 mg. daily doses. Potassium can be taken
in doses of 100 mgs. per day.

• *Zinc* is essential in boosting immune function, which is suppressed
by the stress of anxiety. (Zinc is so essential to the immune system
that many people find it a fast and effective cold-relief remedy, as
well.) This important trace mineral can be taken in 50 mg. doses.

From the Vitamin Shelf

• *The Antioxidants Vitamins A, C, and E.* Antioxidants are substances that bond with "free radicals"—the worn-out cells and

genes adrift in our bloodstream that need to be removed from our bodies. Antioxidants help remove them before they damage still-healthy cells, and so they contribute greatly to immune functioning. Here's the connection to anxiety: When anxiety stresses the body, immune functioning is suppressed. Therefore antioxidant supplementation is recommended.

Vitamin A is a potent ally when anxiety wears us down. Unlike the other antioxidants, however, A is a fat-soluble substance, which means it stores up in the body's fat tissues. High doses, taken over a short period of time, can have a toxic effect. Follow the manufacturers' directions carefully.

Vitamin C. Under stress, our body rapidly loses stores of vitamin C. This vitamin is essential to adrenal-gland functioning—and the adrenals produce the anti-stress hormones we need to keep the physical symptoms of anxiety from taking a terrible toll on our bodies. For this reason, vitamin C supplementation is essential when we're experiencing chronic or extreme anxiety. Vitamin C with *bioflavanoids* is recommended. (See below.) Doses of up to 10,000 mgs. daily can be taken in extreme situations, but doses of 1,000 to 3,000 mgs. daily is the recommended range. When taking this supplement in higher doses, you should drink a minimum of 16 ounces of water to prevent the formation of kidney stones.

Vitamin E. With the immune system embattled during bouts of anxiety, vitamin E is another important antioxidant. It protects cell membranes from free radicals and other damage, which helps our cells use nutrients, thus helping to restore physical energy drained by anxious stress.

• *Vitamin B-Complex.* This family of vitamins is crucial in supporting a wide range of important body functions. When the stress of physical, mental, or spiritual anxiety hits, B vitamins are quickly depleted from the body. Taken together, the B-Complex vitamins have an overall tonic effect, boosting our energy levels by helping our bodies use food-fuel efficiently. Vitamin B-5 (pantothenic acid) is perhaps the most important single B vitamin when we are suffering from anxiety. B-Complex can be taken in relatively high doses because it is water soluble and quickly flushes out of the body, but doses of 100 mg. daily are recommended. B-5 can be taken in doses of 100 mg. up to three times a day. In cases of severe anxiety and physical depletion, a physician may opt to give intra-muscular injections of B-Complex.

Note: Some people are sensitive to B-3 (niacin/naicinimide) and experience a "niacin flush"—including reddened skin, particularly on the upper body, neck, and face, and tingling. Generally, this occurs when taking B-3 in higher doses. As with any reaction, notify your physician if this occurs. Normally, the "niacin flush" is harmless and passes quickly. Drinking several 8-ounce glasses of water helps the symptoms to ease.

• *Bioflavanoids*...otherwise known as *Vitamin P,* are water-soluble antioxidants that greatly enhance the body's absorption and use of vitamin C. For this reason, they're often sold in combination. Derived from fruit and vegetable sources, bioflavanoids may also appear on supplement labels under their individual names, which include *citrin, flavones, flavanols, hesperidin, quercitin,* and *rutin.*

The ABCs (and More)
of Taking Supplements

When you make natural supplements part of your anxiety-relief strategy, there are a few guidelines you need to know. These are simple, but important.

Always discuss the supplements you're taking with your physician. You want to take supplements to enhance, and never to counteract, the effectiveness of other treatments you're receiving from a healthcare professional. Therefore, always disclose your usage of natural supplements.

Buy quality. Just because a supplement is more expensive, doesn't mean it's more potent or effective. Go to websites, and seek information from organizations that test and rate supplements. Check out the product you're buying and its manufacturer. (See "Buying High-Quality Supplements" mentioned earlier in this chapter.)

Carefully read the labels. Some substances are best taken with food. Others are effective when taken in several doses, at different times of day. Many manufacturers will list drugs and other supplements with which their product will have a negative reaction. And, of course, the label will give you the recommended daily dosage, if one has been established.

Give supplements time to work. Even though supplements are potent, it takes time before their effectiveness is evident. Don't expect them to work as quickly as pharmaceuticals. Because it takes longer for a natural substance to build up to a therapeutic level in your body, it can take between two to four weeks before you feel a difference.

Increase your intake of water. It's very important to increase your intake of fluids—particularly water—when taking supplements. Taking a few sips to get the capsules down is not enough. Taking supplements will cause your kidneys and liver to work harder, and water will keep these vital organs flushed and working well. If you are taking higher doses, or taking several supplements, your liver and kidneys most definitely need more water to help them out.

Drink a minimum of four 8-ounce glasses of water a day, and build up to eight glasses if possible. Cool, not cold, water is best.

When taking herbs, more is not better. Some vitamins and minerals are more effective when taken in higher doses. This is not true with herbs. Their effectiveness comes as the therapeutic level *builds* in your body over time. Increasing the dose is generally a waste, and with some herbs it can create toxicity.

Unless you are under the care of a healthcare professional who is trained in the use of herbs, stick with the manufacturers' recommendations.

8

Creating a Balanced Life

*T*oday, the healthcare community is discovering that treating the *whole person* is the best approach to any health condition. Every aspect of our being can, and usually does, contribute to our problems. For that reason, we need to take in the needs of body, mind, and spirit if we want to manage—and cure—any disorder or illness.

The problem is, each healthcare discipline takes its own approach to treating a given health-related problem. So, unfortunately, much as there is agreement that the whole-person approach is best, few are offering the balanced approach that meets the needs of body, mind, and spirit.

Throughout this book we've looked at self-care strategies you can use, combining them with professional advice and support, to relieve anxiety, panic attacks, and anxiety disorders. Finding what works for you is not difficult, but it takes time and requires that you pay attention to what really goes on in *you*.

Learning About You

Understanding ourselves and how we react to life is an art many of us have to learn. The truth is, we all need a bit of help when it comes to really knowing ourselves and learning how we tick.

What follows is a simple tool you can use to build your own self-care plan. *Use* this tool to help you to build a real, whole-person strategy that works to fill your needs...and to help you with that wonder-working thing called *follow-through*.

.so often, we focus on only one area of need—say, the need to .place negative, anxiety-inducing thoughts—and we overlook other areas of need vital to restoring well-being. (If you guessed that getting regular, physical activity is generally the area *most* of us ignore, you'd be exactly right.)

Sometimes, too, we *think* we're doing well in a particular area, but we're not. Again, let's say we recognize our need to replace anxiety-producing thoughts with a positive and healthy thought-flow. We see the need. We tell our closest friends what we've discovered. We even catch and reverse those triggering thoughts and thought-patterns a few times. But the fact is, it takes time to redirect those deep-driving forces at work in our lives. And when we need to repattern several aspects of our life, *we need to give ourselves the grace of a lot of self-support*…along with our commitment and time.

This simple tool will help you with the self-support. (You supply the commitment and time.)

A Healing Journal

You may wish to make copies of the following pages and create a "Healing Journal" by keeping them in a notebook. Use them to record the strategies that work for you, as you build a personalized plan for balanced living.

A few simple instructions will help you use this journal effectively:

- **Every month, choose two anxiety-relief strategies to practice each week.** Use other strategies as you need them, but practice at least two each week.

- **Choose one strategy that helps you challenge anxiety…balanced by one strategy that distracts and relaxes you.** Any time we want to grow and change, we need to both challenge obstacles…and rest from challenge. Being direct and aggressive helps "break down" anxious habits over time; taking the indirect and passive approach "softens" and melts them.

• **Choose a specific time of day. Make it "sacred."** Give yourself enough time every day—*beginning with a minimum of 45 minutes*—to get alone and give focused attention to calming your anxious thoughts and thought patterns. Only *you* will know "how much time" you really require for these practices: The presence of tension…or relaxation…in your own body will be the barometer that tells you. The point is to practice until you can allow a sense of peace to flow throughout your whole being at will.

• **Make notes to yourself about your experience.** These will help you, whether you continue working on your own or seek help from a professional.

In time, you'll want to open up more time into your life for these refreshing activities. And you'll find you're able to use these healthful strategies any time, anywhere.

Calming My Mind

Month: _____

Time: _____

Week 1

Healthy Challenge: _____

Healthy Distraction: _____

Week 2

Healthy Challenge: _____

Healthy Distraction: _____

Week 3

Healthy Challenge: _____

Healthy Distraction: _____

Week 4

Healthy Challenge: _____

Healthy Distraction: _____

Notes

• Anxiety-triggering thoughts and thought patterns I recognize.

_____

_____

_____

• Strategies that relieve mental anxiety.

_____

_____

• Greatest mental challenges. (Thinking that still gets me stuck.)

_____

_____

_____

_____

_____

_____

_____

_____

_____

Lifting My Spirit

Month: _____

Time: _____

Week 1

Healthy Challenge: _____

Healthy Distraction: _____

Week 2

Healthy Challenge: _____

Healthy Distraction: _____

Week 3

Healthy Challenge: _____

Healthy Distraction: _____

Week 4

Healthy Challenge: _____

Healthy Distraction: _____

Notes

• Spiritual values, or beliefs, with which I find myself in tension.

_____

_____

_____

• Strategies that relieve anxiety.

_____

_____

• Greatest spiritual challenges. (Values or beliefs still causing me conflict.)

_____

_____

_____

_____

_____

_____

_____

_____

_____

Mindful and Peaceful Eating Habits
A Transitional Plan

Month: _____

For every elimination add a positive and healthful replacement. (For instance if you eliminate caffeinated hot drinks, replacing coffee with noncaffeinated herbal teas can help with the transition.)

Weeks 1 and 2 Changes

Eliminate: _____

Replacement: _____

Circumstances:
　　　Time(s) of Day: _____

　　　Emotional Atmosphere: _____

　　　Other : _____

Weeks 3 and 4 Changes

Eliminate: _____

Replacement: _____

Circumstances:
　　　Time(s) of Day: _____

　　　Emotional Atmosphere: _____

　　　Other: _____

Notes

• Eliminating/replacing these foods eased physical tension, helped decrease anxiety, and/or helped my digestion.

_____

_____

_____

_____

_____

_____

• Changing certain circumstances that affect my eating/eating habits was helpful/not helpful.

_____

_____

_____

_____

_____

_____

_____

Positively Directed Physical Energy

Month: _____

Time: _____ _____ **times a week**

(Plan for a minimum of two workouts each week, and a day of rest.)

Week 1

Low-Intensity Workout: _____
Moderate-Intensity Workout: _____
Intense Workout: _____
Fun Activity: _____
Day of Rest: _____

Week 2

Low-Intensity Workout: _____
Moderate-Intensity Workout: _____
Intense Workout: _____
Fun Activity: _____
Day of Rest: _____

Week 3

Low-Intensity Workout: _____
Moderate-Intensity Workout: _____
Intense Workout: _____
Fun Activity: _____
Day of Rest: _____

Week 4

Low-Intensity Workout: _____
Moderate-Intensity Workout: _____
Intense Workout: _____
Fun Activity: _____
Day of Rest: _____

Notes

• Heart rate at rest…and during exercise.

_____

• Strategies that distracted and relaxed me.

_____

• Strategies I enjoyed.

_____

• Observations about my sleeping and resting habits.

_____

_____

_____

_____

_____

_____

_____

_____

Natural Supplememnts
(30-Day Trials)

Month: _____

Supplement(s):

_____

_____

Daily/As Needed Dosage: _____

Desired Effect: _____

Medicines/Other Supplements to Avoid:

_____

_____

Week 1

    Observations: _____

Week 2

    Observations: _____

Week 3

    Observations: _____

Week 4

    Observations: _____

Notes

• Taking these supplements helps/does not help me.

_____

_____

_____

_____

_____

_____

• I experience these positive/negative reactions when I take these supplements.

_____

_____

_____

_____

_____

_____

_____

_____

In Closing

My great wish for everyone reading this book is that you'll take charge of your own self-care and find the strategies that help you relieve anxiety. I am confident that, as you *practice* these healthy new inner and outer habits they'll increase the effectiveness of any work you do in conjunction with professional healers.

I also wish you peace, health in balance, and the freedom to live your life at ease again.

The New Nature Institute

The *New Nature Institute* was founded in 1999 for the purpose of exploring the connection between personal health and wellness and spirituality, with the Hebrew-Christian tradition as its spiritual foundation.

Drawing upon this tradition, the Institute supports the belief that humankind is created in the image of God. We are each body, mind, and spirit, and so intricately connected that each aspect of our being affects the others. If one aspect suffers, our whole being suffers; if all aspects are being supported, we will enjoy a greater sense of well-being.

For this reason, the Institute engages in ongoing research in order to provide up-to-date information that supports a "whole person" approach to wellness. Most especially, research is focused on the natural approaches to wellness that support health and vitality in the body, mind, and spirit.

Healthy Body, Healthy Soul is a series of books intended to complement treatment plans provided by healthcare professionals. They are not meant to be used in place of professional consultations and/or treatment plans.

Along with creating written materials, the New Nature Institute also presents seminars, workshops, and retreats on a range of topics relating to spirituality and wellness. These can be tailored for corporate, spiritual community, or general community settings.

For information contact:

David Hazard
The New Nature Institute
P.O. Box 568
Round Hill, Virginia 20142

(540) 338-7032
Exangelos@aol.com

Look for these other books in the
Healthy Body, Healthy Soul series
from Harvest House™ Publishers

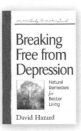

Breaking Free from Depression

Discover how good life is! Based on the idea that spiritual health is the first step to good mental health, this book offers remedies and techniques for overcoming depression.

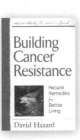

Building Cancer Resistance

Discover simple ways to boost your immune system's resistance to cancer. Based on his premise that a healthy soul contributes to a healthy body, David offers wise suggestions and natural remedies to equip you in the fight for good health.

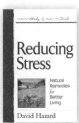

Reducing Stress

People seeking natural ways to combat stress will welcome the commonsense suggestions and simple techniques outlined in this book, written from a unique Christian perspective. Offers tips on everything from relaxation to choosing herb teas.

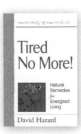

Tired No More!

Tired No More! offers natural energy-boosting strategies anyone can use any time, anywhere, to restore vitality and joy to life. David adds a unique Christian perspective as he emphasizes the importance of good spiritual health in maintaining physical and emotional wellness.